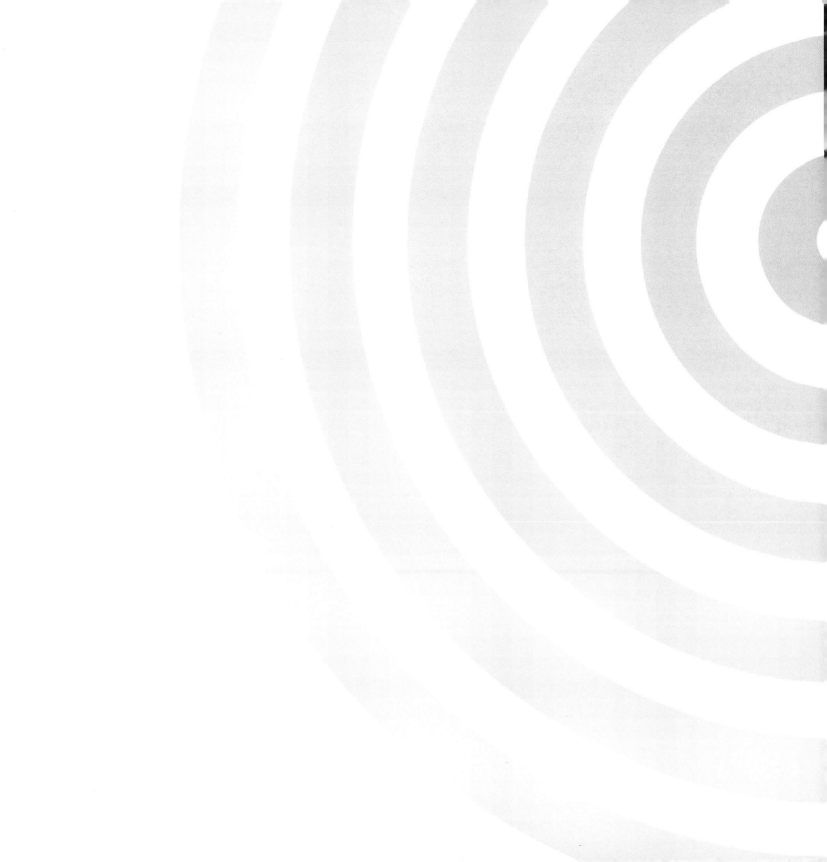

Up Against the Wall

Art, Activism, and the AIDS Poster

Edited by
Donald Albrecht and
Jessica Lacher-Feldman

Medical and Consulting Editor
William M. Valenti, M.D.

RIT Press
Rochester, NY

This book is dedicated to the memory, vision, and passion of Dr. Edward Atwater, and to his wife Ruth, without whom this book and this project would not be possible.

Contents

Foreword

Jonathan P. Binstock and Mary Ann Mavrinac

Up Against the Wall: Art, Activism, and the AIDS Poster is the first major exhibition and accompanying publication devoted to the University of Rochester's collection of AIDS education posters. Organized by the University's Memorial Art Gallery (MAG) in partnership with its River Campus Libraries (RCL), the exhibition and book draw on the RCL's vast collection of HIV/AIDS-related posters held by the Department of Rare Books, Special Collections, and Preservation. The project is timed to open at a critical crossroads in HIV/AIDS funding and advocacy in New York state. Sharing these posters with the Rochester community and beyond is an important priority for MAG and RCL; the exhibition and book also align closely with the larger mission of the University to serve the local community by enhancing public health through the dissemination of fundamental information about HIV/AIDS regionally, nationally, and globally.

This major collaborative project brings together two cultural divisions of the University with a number of key community organizations, such as Trillium Health (a major local healthcare organization founded in the late 1980s as a groundbreaking resource for HIV/AIDS care); Out Alliance (the regional LGBTQ+ community organization in Rochester and one of the oldest in the country); and the Central Library of Rochester and Monroe County. Because of the extraordinary complexity of the project, the team invited key stakeholders, community leaders, and national figures to form an advisory board to help guide the project and build a network of additional stakeholders, potential visitors, sponsors, and donors. The members of the advisory board create a diverse group of partners representative of the larger community, including individuals from arts, healthcare, advocacy, political, community, educational, and faith organizations to help shape this important project. Our collective aim is to heighten awareness about the current state of HIV/AIDS, and to engage the broader community in discourse about a topic many still consider controversial and sensitive, with a goal of fostering lifelong learning. *The AIDS crisis isn't over.* We are in the midst of the AIDS pandemic. However, for many people, it is not part of their sphere. Yet the history of this ongoing crisis, dating from the early 1980s, affects us all.

Monroe County, in which the City of Rochester lies, has the state's second-highest rate of infection outside of New York City, a rate that has increased dramatically over the last five years. In addition, the growing opioid crisis in this community increases the risks of HIV infection. Ending the AIDS epidemic in New York state is an important goal for Governor Andrew Cuomo, who has laid out a plan to reduce the number of new HIV infections, achieving the first-ever decrease in HIV prevalence in the state. This project is timely and essential, as it will heighten awareness about the current state of the AIDS crisis and educate this community about HIV/AIDS prevention, the risks related to exposure, treatment options, and the need for a better understanding of disease prevention.

Donated to the University by physician and medical historian Dr. Edward C. Atwater (1926–2019), the AIDS poster collection is one of the largest of its kind in the world, documenting and illustrating the efforts of various individuals, groups, and organizations, as well as their agendas and missions, to educate and inform the population about HIV/AIDS. The scope of the collection is vast, currently encompassing more than 8,000 posters. Its connection to social and cultural history is palpable. The messages depicted in the posters represent and illustrate cultural, political, sexual, and social differences in diverse communities and locations through language, image, and messaging dating from 1982, the very beginnings of the AIDS crisis, through the present day.

The audience for this project could easily be defined as that of "sexual beings." We have identified key stakeholders and audiences for the project that include people who know very little about HIV/AIDS, especially younger people who do not recognize that we are still in the midst of a crisis, as well as those in the community who have experienced the effects of HIV/AIDS in their own circles. Because of the prevalence of HIV/AIDS, we know that these audiences overlap and that the notion of "a general public" includes all of these stakeholders, since without education and prevention, everyone

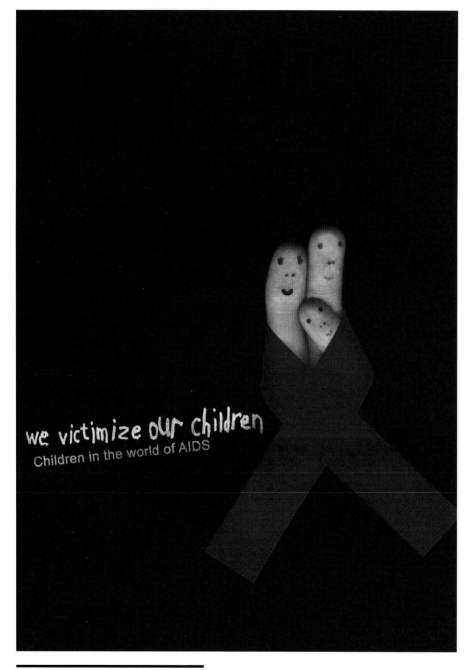

"We Victimize Our Children.
Children in the World of AIDS," 2008
Iran
Designer: Payam Abdolsamadi
102 x 71 cm
AP50033

faces risks. The exhibition and book provide a unique opportunity to inform a broad and diverse audience, from middle-school students through adults of all ages, as well as targeting specific groups through programming, docent tours, and guerrilla marketing. For these audiences, the project has gained special relevance in light of today's COVID-19 pandemic. Too new to write about with the same historical perspective as HIV/AIDS, COVID-19 nonetheless provides a contemporary lens on how visual communications have long been important weapons in the fight against pandemics.

Up Against the Wall is uniquely relevant to Rochester because of this poster collection, but also because Rochester has been at the forefront of HIV/AIDS education and research since the 1980s. The University has a highly ranked medical school conducting important research in infectious diseases including HIV/AIDS. Major discoveries and breakthroughs in such research have taken place in Rochester and by doctors trained at the University, including Dr. Michael Gottlieb, a member of our advisory board, who is best known for his 1981 identification of AIDS as a new disease, as well as for his activism and philanthropic efforts associated with HIV/AIDS treatment.

We wish to thank the many people who have played key roles in this project. Donald Albrecht has served as guest curator of the exhibition and the book's editor, working closely with co-editor and curatorial liaison Jessica Lacher-Feldman, exhibits and special projects manager, RCL, who is the subject specialist and curator of record for the poster collection. The exhibition project is directed by Margot Muto, head of exhibitions at MAG, and supported and executed by a cohesive team working together to assure its success. Other key personnel include Maurini Strub, River Campus Library's director, performance & user engagement; Sheryl Burgstrom, MAG's director of finance; Debra Foster, MAG's director of facilities and security; Siri Baker, MAG's director of advancement; Joseph Carney, senior director of major gifts; Chris Garland, MAG's assistant director of advancement; Pamela Jackson, senior director of advancement for RCL; and Rachael Brown, MAG's director of marketing and engagement. Their work is supported by librarians/archivists, museum staff, and others, making a comprehensive team with a broad range of expertise to support the work of this ambitious and multi-faceted project. We also thank Ian Bradley-Perrin, Ph.D. candidate at Columbia University, who developed the extended captions that accompany the posters, and the authors who have contributed to this book. Their work was reviewed and commented upon by Ian Bradley-Perrin, Tamar W. Carroll, and Stephen Vider. We acknowledge the great skill and efforts of the book's publisher, RIT Press at Rochester Institute of Technology: director Bruce Austin, managing editor Molly Cort, designer and marketing specialist Marnie Soom, and business manager Laura DiPonzio Heise.

Finally, we are all indebted to Dr. Atwater. His interest in this project was unwavering until his death in April of 2019, and it has provided us with an inexhaustible source of inspiration throughout the project's progress.

Up Against the Wall provides the Rochester community with an unparalleled range of public programs and innovative marketing that together explore the intersection of art, personal and public health, as well as community dialogue. They also serve as crucial points of engagement. Public programming, community engagement, marketing, and public relations are deeply linked in this project, each informing the others and blending together as the posters lend themselves to a variety of intersectional synergies. Working with focus groups, key community organizations, a community liaison, and volunteers, our goal is to make the exhibition as well as MAG's auditorium and classrooms available to the greater community for programs held in conjunction with the exhibition.

Finally, we are delighted and grateful to acknowledge the project's funders: Vicki and Richard Schwartz, the Rochester Area Community Foundation's Lloyd E. Klos Fund, Friends of the University of Rochester Libraries, DKT International, and the Gleason Family Foundation. Additional support has been provided by the Family of Dr. Edward C. Atwater, Helen H. Berkeley, Canandaigua National Bank and Trust, the Gallery Council of the Memorial Art Gallery, the Anthony J. Mascioli Trust, Suzanne M. Spencer, and an anonymous donor.

Funding is also provided by the Thomas and Marion Hawks Memorial Fund, the Robert L. and Mary L. Sproull Fund, and the Nancy R. Turner Fund for Special Exhibitions.

The exhibition is supported in part by awards from the National Endowment for the Arts and the Institute of Museum and Library Services MA-245369-OMS-20. The views, findings, conclusions or recommendations expressed in this exhibition do not necessarily represent those of the Institute of Museum and Library Services.

The book that complements the exhibition is made possible by William M. Valenti, M.D., who served as medical and consulting editor for the book project.

Preface
Locating AIDS in an Image Commons

Avram Finkelstein

In advertising, ubiquity is a key component to commercial dominance. Unfortunately, marketing dollars alone can't guarantee that a message will capture the zeitgeist, lead to an advertising franchise, or build a legacy brand. The sort of messaging content required for that kind of foothold demands a granular reading of audience and an even deeper reading of social context. Content generates influence, and context transforms it into dominion.

When held up against the social significance of political agency or public health, the kind of sovereignty sought through multinational corporate branding is utterly trivial. Lives do not hang in the balance every time Coca-Cola struggles to reinvent what it already owns. But we live in a culture that revolves around images, and such a culture creates a specific kind of public square, an "image commons," a space in which the same rules apply to social movements as to the marketing of soft drinks.

It's uncomfortable to consider that matters of health and commerce might exist on the same continuum, although the archives of the University of Rochester's AIDS Education Posters collection holds thousands of examples that prove they can. Created over decades and across international borders, the posters each serve as a matrix for reaching audiences with lifesaving information the way advertising does, using vernacular toolboxes of understanding, humor, advocacy, and common sense, to provide bread-crumb trails for future social historians.

But given the expanding emphasis on information technologies and the migration of advertising dollars to digital platforms, some argue the poster is dead, a vestigial signifier of the outmoded physical spaces our new media landscape appears to be kissing goodbye. Perhaps, but we still have bodies, many of which reside in homes, homes on streets, streets we inevitably traverse. Consequently, our corporeality imposes organic limits on the obsolescence of the physical spaces we occupy, and if one needs hard proof of the continued productivity of these shared spaces, our population centers remain flooded with the messaging that sells us everything from goods to celebrities, from politicians to personal identity. Virtual advertising spaces continue to evolve, but our physical commons is still thriving as well.

Moreover, the commercial and institutional enterprises that commit marketing dollars to these spaces still subscribe to the poster as a viable format, declaring it very much alive. As a means of communication, the poster is pretty hard to argue against: it is direct, visceral, ecomomical, compelling, persuasive, arresting, resourceful, and authentic. It is, and always has been, a marketing workhorse, and we have centuries of evidence of its capacity to winnow the complexities of political agency to the sort of plainspokenness that social movements depend on.

Examples of this capability are frequently drawn from the cultural output associated with ACT UP (AIDS Coalition to Unleash Power) in New York, which thought strategically about its proximity to the media and political centers in eastern America, and is often deployed as a template for how image ecospheres might constitute themselves. To be sure, useful lessons can be found through the study of this cultural production, as typified by the "Silence = Death" poster. But archival finding aids do not help us understand how or why such posters worked and are powerless to untangle the complex web of social context connecting this cultural production to grassroots organizing or to the dissemination of these organizing materials.

For instance, the lack of societal candor about the vastness of human sexuality exacerbated by the rise of the religious right and the deliberate pace of epidemiological analysis were easily fanned into a bonfire by the concomitant deregulation of American media that triggered the 24/7 cable news cycle, an uncharted social landscape at that time. AIDS "storytelling" (as distinct from the story of AIDS) began here, when the sudden spike in airtime made it easy for producers to green-light AIDS content to deliver "information" to panicked audiences who thought they could easily "catch" AIDS from a mosquito bite or a toilet seat. The press was hungry for data and analysis, and ACT UP provided tons of it. When evaluating this body of activist output, one should remember that the phenomenology of the media landscape that proliferated its messaging was specific to it and is irreproducible.

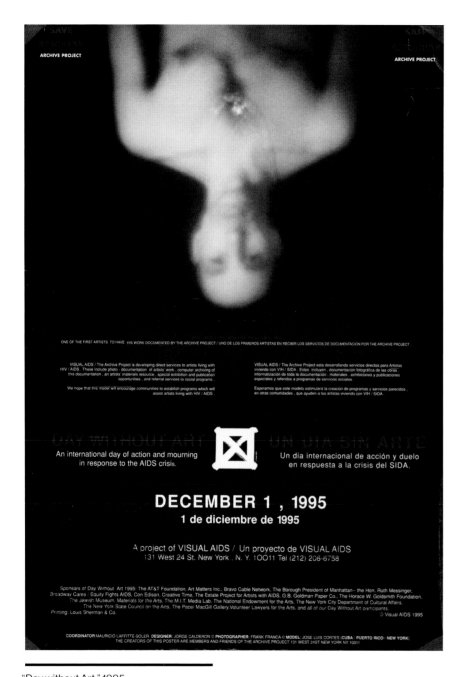

"Day without Art," 1995
Series: *Day without Art*
New York, New York, U.S.A.
Creator: Visual AIDS
Designer: José Luis Cortés
90 x 62 cm
AP5225

Reagan's deregulation-mad America also created tax abatements for Manhattan real estate developers, which led to a building boom that triggered a radical increase in construction sites, which posters needed for their display. This made postering a relatively inexpensive, high-visibility form of mass communication in New York and an essential component of street life. And deregulation fostered a receptivity within the pharmaceutical industry and American research communities for the fast-tracking of the HIV drug development pipeline as well, which was supported in tandem by mediagenic activists, vividly underscoring the promise of a burgeoning marketplace for AIDS drugs.

Images have undeniable power in an image culture and intrinsic significance to curators, historians, and archivists. But archives cannot, in and of themselves, reflect the intricacies of neo-liberalism without the exhaustive research needed to connect all the dots and create meaning from this material. Books, like the one cradled in your hands, become essential components to helping us understand the social use of the story of HIV and AIDS for future activists, culture workers, and students of history.

To create social context for these posters, one needs more comprehensive analytical tools than archival finding aids frequently offer. When it comes to content, however, these posters are able to speak for themselves and remain relevant to twenty-first-century communication strategies. The powerful terseness of the poster is the kissing cousin of the soundbite and the meme. It is an abbreviation of content that maintains both authenticity of format and the kind of vernacular truism we used to refer to as "folk wisdom." Whether the poster exists as a physical object or a download, and our social spaces are actual or virtual, it is the poster's content that tempts us to pass powerful images from hand to hand.

The poster, regardless of delivery system, will never become obsolete. It is the equivalent of the exercise of fabricating a teapot in Japanese ceramic traditions, which is not, in the end, about tea; it is about the performance of the meaningful complexities of collaborative endeavor in shared spaces. Without the collective gestures that lead to the activation of our public sphere, a poster is not worth the paper it is printed on. If, however, it is an exercise in paring communication down to one essential social purpose, that of expressing human care in any of the millions of forms in which humanity articulates its deeper meanings, then the humble poster is without peer and is ensured eternal relevance.

Introduction
A Historical Perspective

Donald Albrecht

In the spring of 1981, the United States Centers for Disease Control and Prevention (CDC) reported on a mysterious infection that caused pneumonia in five young gay men living in Los Angeles. On July 3 of that year, *The New York Times* published its first article on the illness, reporting on 41 infected gay men in New York and California, and publicizing this deadly new disease, a year later termed HIV/AIDS. The disease that press coverage such as the *Times* article initially associated with "others"—gay men and intravenous drug users who were not likely to infect the general public—quickly grew into a widening pandemic, with hundreds, then thousands, and ultimately millions of people affected worldwide. Consider these staggering statistics: since HIV/AIDS was first detected in the early 1980s, an estimated 78 million people have become infected with HIV, and 35 million people have died of AIDS-related illnesses.

In the three-plus decades since the CDC announcement, the public perception and understanding of the HIV/AIDS disease has followed a convoluted trajectory. While the press initially focused on gay men and drug users, as early as 1982 AIDS-related diseases had already affected children and blood transfusion recipients. Since the HIV virus that causes AIDS was not identified until 1983, misinformation about its transmission was widespread, and confusion, panic, and anxiety about causes and carriers continued to grow among at-risk groups as well as the general public. Small organizations of volunteers, notably

New York's Gay Men's Health Crisis, founded in 1982, and the Victorian AIDS Council, started by the Melbourne, Australia, gay community in 1983, were among the first to spring up to educate their communities. By the mid-1980s, however, established public health authorities and national governments recognized that the AIDS pandemic had spread beyond the initially affected groups. President Ronald Reagan first mentioned AIDS publicly in a 1985 press conference. In an acknowledgement of the international scope and scale of the AIDS crisis, the World Health Organization (WHO) founded World AIDS Day, the first-ever global health day, in 1988. By the early 1990s, the introduction of new drug treatments meant the disease was no longer a death sentence. Yet the number of people infected with HIV/AIDS remains high. As of 2018, 37.9 million people worldwide were living with HIV/AIDS, including 1.7 million children younger than 15 years of age, and governments and global organizations continue to face challenges in stopping new infections and making sure that people with the disease receive treatment.

Throughout this period, AIDS activists have spread educational messages to at-risk groups and the general public, often using one of visual culture's least expensive and most ephemeral media: the poster. Working from within small, community protest groups, who were often the first to realize the power of posters, and governmental health departments, activists have created posters that promoted the message of

disease prevention through safer sex, debunked misinformation about HIV/AIDS transmission, and urged compassion for people living with AIDS. Debates and contentious battles have also erupted. Proponents of condoms as the best means of prevention have fought religious groups who are against homosexuality and any form of contraception. Beyond serving as public health communiqués, posters (and related fliers, buttons, and other media) promoted positive messages, urged action (the most famous, perhaps, being the "Silence = Death" poster), and forged identity and community among AIDS activists. HIV/AIDS posters appeared on billboards and buses, queer clubs and doctors' offices.

Posters, with their seamless fusion of text and image, have been well suited to conveying a wide range of messages to a variety of publics. With their international scope, strong messaging, and myriad visual languages—from simple hand drawings to slick advertising graphics—HIV/AIDS posters have revived the genre of the public health poster and represent one of the most significant chapters in the more than 150-year history of poster art. Invented in the early nineteenth century, posters reached their modern form around 1880 with the introduction of a lithographic process, mastered by French artist Jules Chéret, that allowed artists to create rainbow-hued posters by using three stones (red, yellow, blue) in registration. These pioneering posters sold the public popular entertainments such as operas, cabarets, and bullfights, and consumer products from coffee to biscuits.

Posters became truly potent forms of propaganda with the outbreak of World War I in Europe and the United States. They graphically and rhetorically prompted people to hate the enemy, buy war bonds, save food, and enlist in the armed forces. The war also brought about the widespread use of posters for health campaigns to promote nursing, support aid organizations like the American Red Cross, and warn against a slew of maladies. These posters replaced other forms of visual communication, most notably broadsides—large sheets of paper printed only on one side and mainly composed of text—that for centuries had told the public about the threats of, and educated them about the possible cures for, such diseases as plague and cholera.

The capacity of posters to mix text and images made them a powerful and persuasive means of communicating information about a wide range of diseases and health issues throughout the twentieth century. Since early in the century, health posters have addressed tuberculosis, the first infectious disease to spark nationally coordinated campaigns stressing possible recovery through rest, fresh air, and a healthy diet. Governments targeted the scourge of venereal diseases and the need for sexual abstention or condoms during both World War I and World War II. Posters have also warned of threats to the public exposed to environmental

hazards such as air pollution, asbestos, and lead paint, emphasizing responsible actions to combat them via individual, government, and corporate responses. Starting in the 1960s, health campaigns have fought against cigarettes as a cause of cancer, cautioning people about the hazards of smoking.

The advent of HIV/AIDS in the early 1980s offered new and different challenges to health poster sponsors and designers. Unlike other sexually transmitted diseases such as syphilis and gonorrhea, the existence of which had been known for centuries, the unexpectedly rapid spread of HIV/AIDS from the early 1980s on, the widespread confusion over its transmission, and the early realization that the disease was international in scope fostered the production of thousands of posters in 100-plus countries worldwide. At the same time, AIDS put differences in gender, sexuality, and other factors into sharp relief, and the diversity of those affected— men, women, and children; homosexuals and heterosexuals; individuals and families; drug users and sex workers—multiplied the number of posters targeting specific audiences.

At the same time, the international reach of the disease prompted diverse visual iconography and design styles attuned to the cultural conditions of different countries where posters were produced. "In the West," notes design historian Steven Heller, "AIDS posters polemically attack the issue, yet in India, for instance, they more touchingly convey stories designed as

warnings to alter common behavior... [and use] vernacular imagery rendered in popular styles" such as drawings of men and women dressed in brightly colored and patterned clothes.[1] Such simple, yet colorful, drawings of people also have characterized HIV/AIDS posters promoting safer sex in most African nations, where AIDS is prevalent among heterosexuals.

Even within the West, however, approaches to HIV/AIDS posters have varied. Dr. Edward C. Atwater, whose collection this publication and related exhibition celebrate, noted that, in general, posters issued by the American government were not that visually striking "because they had to be neutral. They had to be careful not to offend some group or some sensibility so the best American posters were usually put up by private organizations... But in Iceland, they had a couple posters with dozens of prominent entertainers and political figures doing something silly with a condom. Can you imagine Barbara Bush doing something silly with a condom on a poster? It shows what people in Iceland were willing to do [for the cause] that people here I don't think were willing to do."[2]

In their search for visual iconography, HIV/AIDS health poster sponsors and designers found inspiration in historical public health examples. Their messaging assumed a variety of forms that HIV/AIDS posters also adopted. They sought to educate people about how to recognize a disease's symptoms so they would

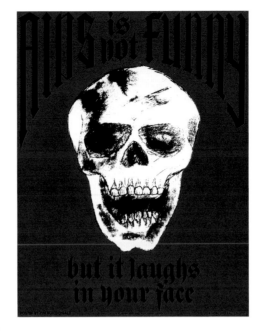

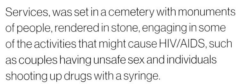

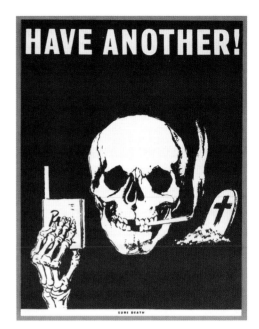

seek treatment. They advocated behavior that wouldn't transmit the disease to others. They also encouraged compassion for those infected, and, more generally, linked health to patriotism and good moral behavior.

The oldest visual tradition that HIV/AIDS posters have drawn upon was far older than poster art itself. Specters of death and decay—skulls, skeletons, and graveyards—have been prevalent symbols of mortality in art and literature for centuries, from Hamlet's meditation on Yorick's skull to Mexican Day of the Dead imagery. Skulls also appeared in some of the earliest French health posters of the first decades of the twentieth century. This deadly imagery sought to warn against the fatal consequences (and the need for awareness and prevention) of venereal diseases during World War I, and continued to be deployed for similar campaigns during World War II. It was also used in postwar anti-cigarette campaigns; one particularly ominous poster depicted a smoking skull with the text "Sure Death."

HIV/AIDS posters adopted this imagery in a variety of ways. Morgue images, for instance, have frequently been used to advise people against risky behavior. One poster depicted a morgue slab on which lay a corpse, its big toe tagged "AIDS." Another morgue image wryly admonished, "Don't Let Love Sweep You off Your Feet." A poster of a grimacing skull announced, "AIDS Is Not Funny but It Laughs in Your Face." One poster series, produced by a Québec advertising agency for the Ministry of Health and Social

Services, was set in a cemetery with monuments of people, rendered in stone, engaging in some of the activities that might cause HIV/AIDS, such as couples having unsafe sex and individuals shooting up drugs with a syringe.

HIV/AIDS posters that used scare tactics not only harkened back to the morbid imagery of previous health posters, but also perpetuated their phobias against certain people: wartime posters about venereal diseases, for example, singled out women as guilty culprits and men as innocent victims deserving protection, although, in reality, both were equal partners. HIV/AIDS posters with images of death and contagion might similarly stigmatize people with the disease. In a text written for this book, Ken Monteith, executive director of COCQ-SIDA (Coalition des organismes communautaires québécois de lutte contre le SIDA), notes that the death message of the Ministry of Health and Social Services' cemetery monument posters "couldn't have been clearer, or more rejected by, the community of people living with HIV." At the same time, Monteith's organization, which sought to integrate people with AIDS into their communities, distributed a poster that depicted

a man and a woman asleep in a coffin, with the tagline "AIDS Does Not Forgive." The poster, he writes, "reinforced the 'death' message and further stymied the fight for inclusion." (The poster, created by an ad agency, convinced Monteith's organization not to accept such campaigns without playing a part in their creation.)

While overt icons of death and decay such as skulls, coffins, and cemeteries have made frequent appearances in the visual repertoire of public health posters, their opposite—vibrant and healthy bodies—have also been prevalent. This visual trope has been employed to suggest that in some cases good looks can be deceiving. Many posters have deployed images of seemingly healthy people who are unaware that they have a disease or who may transmit the disease to unsuspecting people. These messages have prompted people to get tested and, in the case of venereal diseases, to beware of having sex with those who might have such diseases but don't look like they do. "'Healthy Looks' Can Hide Tuberculosis," proclaimed a 1930s American poster, "the X-ray Will Show It before *You* Know It." Anti-venereal disease posters often featured portraits of a seemingly

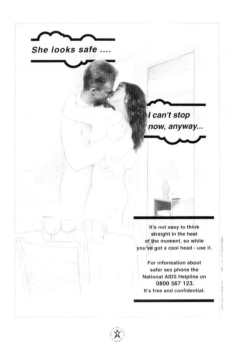

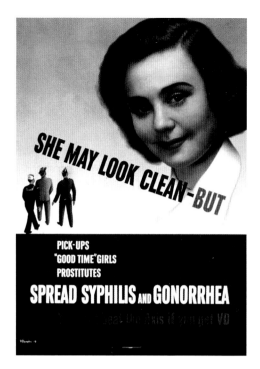

"She Looks Safe....
I Can't Stop Now Anyway..." 1992
London, England, UK
Creator: Health Education Authority
60 x 42 cm
AP6107

"She May Look Clean—But Pick-ups,
'Good Time' Girls, Prostitutes Spread
Syphilis and Gonorrhea," ca. 1940
U.S.A.
Creator: U.S. Government
National Institutes of Health

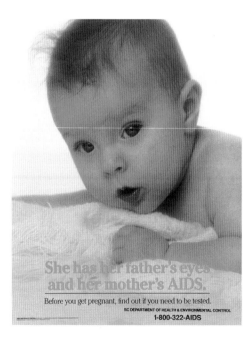

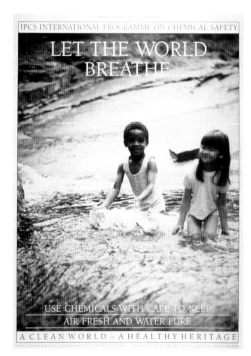

"She Has Her Father's Eyes
and Her Mother's AIDS," 1988
South Carolina, U.S.A
Creator: South Carolina Department of
Health and Environmental Control
61 x 46 cm
AP1631

"Let the World Breathe," ca. 1984
Geneva, Switzerland
Creator: International Programme on
Chemical Safety and World Health
Organization
World Health Organization
via National Institutes of Health

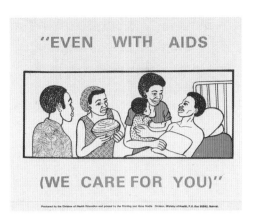

"Even with AIDS (We Care for You)," n.d.
Nairobi, Kenya
Creator: National AIDS and
STDs Control Programme
34 x 46 cm
AP3456

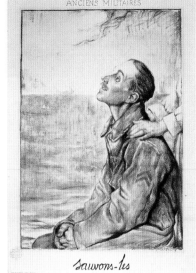

"National Day of Tuberculosis.
Former Soldiers: Save Them"
(translated from French), 1919
France
Creator: Journée Nationale
des Tuberculeux
Designer: Abel Faivre
National Institutes of Health

healthy "girl next door" as a warning: "She May Look Clean," an American World War II poster announced, "But Pick-ups, 'Good Time' Girls, Prostitutes Spread Syphilis and Gonorrhea." Extending these visual themes into the arena of HIV/AIDS, a Canadian poster proclaimed, "Looks Can Be Deceiving" above a photograph of a healthy family. The Centers for Disease Control produced a poster of a smiling, beautiful woman: "She Shows All the Signs of Having HIV. *There Aren't Any You Can See.* You Just Can't Tell from Outward Appearance..." Unprotected sex can also have unintended and deadly consequences. "She Looks Safe..." thought a man in a British poster embracing a woman—perpetuating the historic notion of women as carriers of venereal disease—as she acknowledged, "I Can't Stop Now, Anyway...". The poster exhorted, "It's Not Easy to Think Straight in the Heat of the Moment, So While You've Got a Cool Head—Use It."

Another popular public health message has focused on the need to protect the innocent victims of a disease. Educational campaigns about the negative effects of smoking, air pollution, and lead paint often used the imagery of children, pregnant women, and families, aiming to convince adults and policy makers to act responsibly in order not to affect the healthy with their actions. Similarly, an HIV/AIDS poster of a baby states, "She Has Her Father's Eyes and Her Mother's AIDS."

Public health posters have endorsed compassion for the people infected with the disease with images of them being cared for or asking to be cared for by healthy people. Historical precedents included a ca. 1919 poster in which the hand of someone outside the poster's edge rests on the shoulder of a tuberculosis victim to comfort him. Fighting for AIDS patients, a 1987 poster, rendered as a stick-figure drawing, showed a child crying "I Have AIDS. Please Hug Me. I Can't Make You Sick." This poster was most likely sparked by debates between parents, teachers, and school boards over admitting or excluding children with AIDS from schools. Circulating around this time was a widely publicized example of this debate: the story of Indiana teenager Ryan White, who contracted AIDS as a hemophiliac and was denied access to high school until a court order ruled in his favor.

More visually sophisticated was the poster created for Italian clothing company Benetton that evoked the image of the dying Christ in its photograph of a young man, his body ravaged by AIDS, on his deathbed, surrounded by his distraught family whose embraces comfort him and each other. As in the 1919 poster, the hand of a caregiver, named Peta, reaches out to the dying man. "Let Peta's wrist—and spirit," notes writer, activist, and artist Theodore Kerr in this book, "encourage viewers to look beyond the poster frame, searching for the stories untold, and the context needed to better understand the history and ongoingness of HIV/AIDS."

Erroneous fears of infection simply by being close to people with AIDS and breathing the same air fostered some of the most poignant posters goading their viewers to understand and show empathy for people with HIV/AIDS. Characteristic of the straightforward posters coming out of Africa, an example from Ghana depicted a woman spoon-feeding a bedridden man with a simple message, "Give People with AIDS Love and Care." Posters such as these have aimed to transform misperceptions about HIV/AIDS and its victims.

Given the seriousness of the health poster's subject matter, it may seem surprising that designers have wielded humor or visual puns to convince people to take action against a disease. A 1943 World War II poster about venereal disease, for example, punned that its unsuspecting soldier "'Picked up' More Than a Girl" by hiring a sex worker. This strategy worked to catch the

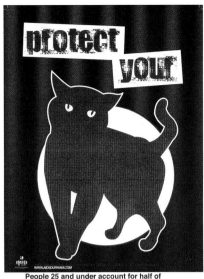

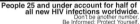

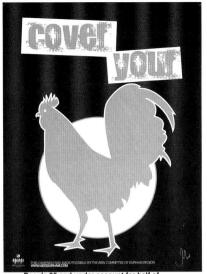

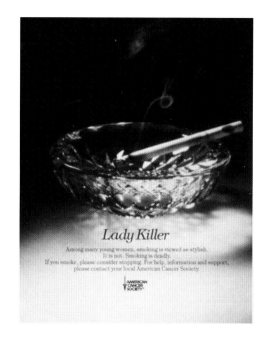

"Protect Your [Pussy]," 2010
Oshawa, Ontario, Canada
Creator: AIDS Committee of Durham Region
Designer: Youth for Youth
28 x 19 cm
AP9001

"Cover Your [Cock]," 2010
Oshawa, Ontario, Canada
Creator: AIDS Committee of Durham Region
Designer: Youth for Youth
28 x 19 cm
AP9000

viewers' attention, with the intent to make them stop, think, and do a double take.

Some HIV/AIDS posters have also used this approach. Over a colorful painting of a man and a woman locked in a sexual position in the style of the Hindu Kama Sutra, for example, an American poster noted, "If You Think This Looks Dangerous, Try Doing It without a Condom." Similarly, a pair of Canadian posters punned on slang expressions for female and male genitalia, picturing a pink cat and a blue rooster to visually complete the

sentences, "Protect Your..." and "Cover Your...". Noting that thousands of young people die in car accidents caused by drugs and alcohol but that having risky sex can also kill by transmitting AIDS, a poster for the American National Institute on Drug Abuse combined a photograph of a young woman and man kissing in a car with the admonishment that "Vanessa Was In a Fatal Car Accident Last Night. Only She Doesn't Know It Yet."

While HIV/AIDS posters have often built on the visual traditions of health posters, they also radically departed from that history, most notably in the HIV/AIDS posters' overt depictions of nude bodies, sexual intercourse, and condoms. Previous posters that warned against sexually transmitted diseases, most notably those created in the early twentieth century, adhered to Victorian-era attitudes of abstention—an anti-sex position manifested in World War I and II posters. In contrast, HIV/AIDS posters developed in the 1980s—two decades after the sexual revolution in the West—have included images of people, most notably gay men and lesbians, engaging in "safe sex" promoting the message that pleasurable sex is possible without transmitting HIV/AIDS. The Safe Sex Is Hot

Sex campaign by Red Hot Organization in New York, for example, depicted various nude couples in sexual acts.

But perhaps no aspect of HIV/AIDS posters has defined their difference from previous health posters more than their close association with homosexuality. Marginalized and often vilified, gay men were the disease's first and most visible victims—and to some they were the culprits who spread it. In response to their ostracization, gay men formed their own collectives to take action, often producing posters as part of their campaigns. Posters encouraging condom use proliferated with homoerotic imagery of unprecedented frankness, attuned to the work of such celebrated photographers as Robert Mapplethorpe. Exhibited and published as fine art, his erotic photographs examined a wide range of sexual subjects, including male nudes and the sadomasochistic subculture of 1970s New York. Other posters took on government inaction, including, for instance, ones that plastered the words "AIDSGATE" and "He Kills Me" below the face of President Ronald Reagan, who didn't mention AIDS publicly until 1985, after thousands of Americans had already died of the disease. As scholar Tamar W. Carroll has noted in her book *Mobilizing New York*, some of these posters drew on feminist art, specifically the work of Barbara Kruger. The boldface type treatment adopted by some AIDS activists picked up on Kruger's "dramatic poster artwork," according to Carroll, that "sought to hold the art world accountable for its depiction of women as sexual objects and for its dismissal of work by female artists."[3]

HIV/AIDS posters that illustrated condoms were prevalent, especially after the mid-1980s when medical and health experts, from American surgeon general C. Everett Koop to the World Health Organization, supported condoms as the best and safest method to stop the spread of the disease. While previous health poster campaigns against venereal diseases focused on images of potential carriers such as femme-fatale-like prostitutes, HIV/AIDS posters have shown the condom itself in a wide array of guises: photographs of condoms on erect penises and drawings of condoms as fashion accessories ("These Go with Everything!") coming out of gay-friendly San Francisco, collages of condoms being passed between man and God in Michelangelo's Sistine Chapel fresco in Brazil, and even condoms representing the letter "O" in a series of Swiss posters announcing bravO, Ok, and tOnight with the tagline "Stop AIDS." Condoms have appeared as cute and animated cartoon characters, and a campaign featuring a character named Condoman

targeted Aboriginal men in Australia, for whom wearing a condom was often a cultural stigma. This diversity of design expression supports theorist Paula A. Treichler's contention that while HIV/AIDS health posters promoting condoms follow "generic templates," those created "on the ground" are more likely to embrace a country's cultural norms—"a strategy that could be called 'think globally, fuck locally.'"[4]

Today, the poster still plays a role in HIV awareness and prevention, but its messages, imagery, and delivery systems have changed with the times. Contemporary posters promote the most up-to-date science to an audience that has been surrounded by HIV/AIDS messaging for decades, and for whom the disease is no longer a near-certain death sentence but a manageable chronic condition.[5] At the same time, posters based on the imagery and rhetoric of fear and scare tactics have largely disappeared. Sexuality and sexual differences are depicted more openly than ever, and campaigns urging personal responsibility such as "HIV Stops with Me" focus on the faces of HIV-positive people. Changes in messaging and imagery have been matched by transformations in how people encounter HIV posters. Still seen on the street and subway, posters now freely circulate on websites and social media and pop up on smartphones and mobile devices. HIV poster-making will thus continue. HIV posters will morph in lockstep with medical advances and knowledge and perceptions of HIV until the disease is eliminated.

At that hoped-for time, the HIV poster will enter the history books—a dynamic chapter in the trajectory of the health poster, both building on tradition and adding to it in creative ways.

Notes

1. Steven Heller, "Tough, Durable, and Informative: Posters in the Age of HIV/AIDS," in *Graphic Intervention: 25 Years of International AIDS Awareness Posters, 1985–2010*, ed. Javier Cortés and Elizabeth Resnick (Boston, MA: Massachusetts College of Art and Design, 2010), 9.

2. Edward C. Atwater, quoted in Hans Villarica, "30 Years of AIDS," *The Atlantic*, (November 30, 2011), https://www.theatlantic.com/health/archive/2011/11/30-years-of-aids-6-200-iconic-posters-100-countries-1-collector/248737/ (accessed February 24, 2019).

3. Tamar W. Carroll, *Mobilizing New York: AIDS, Antipoverty, and Feminist Activism* (Chapel Hill, NC: The University of North Carolina Press, 2015), 137.

4. Paula A. Treichler, *How to Have Theory in an Epidemic: Cultural Chronicles of AIDS* (Durham, NC: Duke University Press, 1999), 228.

5. Messages urge the use of PrEP (Pre-Exposure Prophylaxis), a preventative medicine for people with a high risk of getting HIV, and support concepts like U = U (Undetectable = Untransmittable), which asserts that HIV-positive people with an undetectable amount of the virus in their blood cannot sexually transmit it to others.

Worlds of Signification
Power and Subjectivity in Global AIDS Posters

Jennifer Brier and Matthew Wizinsky

The Unfurling of Multiple Epidemics

We all live with AIDS. Some of us live with HIV, the virus that causes AIDS, in our bodies. We face attempts to control and surveil our actions and behaviors. We sometimes receive care and treatment for how the disease affects us. Some of us live with AIDS outside our bodies. We experience the cultural and sexual effects of AIDS, whether that includes how we navigate healthcare systems or conceive of and negotiate notions of risk. While both groups can, and sometimes do, choose to ignore AIDS, only people who believe they are immune can do so with impunity. The AIDS epidemic has affected, and continues to affect, everyone on the planet. No one has been immune to the seismic social, medical, and political impact of AIDS during the past forty years. We all live with AIDS. We can all fight against AIDS.

The images presented in this book are from a collection of more than 8,000 posters and related ephemera held in the Rare Books and Special Collections, River Campus Libraries at the University of Rochester. The posters are a visual record of the complex ubiquity of AIDS (Acquired Immune Deficiency Syndrome). They produce a kaleidoscope of visual information—moral instructions, prescriptions for imagined and real behaviors, calls to action, identity-making metaphors, cultural markers, and more. As individuals, each poster attempts to describe some aspect of an impossibly sprawling subject and provides a unique and discrete constellation of ideas, metaphors, and cultural encodings. Each poster produces meaning, whether by calling forth new patterns of individual behaviors in the form of "safer sex" or no sex at all, naming "the state" as a key actor in a process of making citizens healthy, generating new metaphors to experience or comprehend AIDS, or imploring direct action and protest in response to AIDS.

Many of these posters were made in the 1980s and '90s, just before the Internet fundamentally changed how we access and understand images. They were designed as physical objects made for physical spaces—on the walls of bars, health clinics, and doctors' offices, and in public spaces such as urban streetscapes, on mass transit, and even pasted on scaffolding marked "post no bills." They were meant to be seen and interpreted in person, at a specific place and time.

Just as no two posters are identical, the AIDS epidemic is multifarious. Studying this collection confirms what cultural theorist Paula Treichler meant when she described AIDS as an "epidemic of signification."[1] In coining this phrase—one that has been taken up in most subsequent historical texts on AIDS—Treichler wanted us to see that "the AIDS epidemic—with its genuine potential for global devastation—is simultaneously an epidemic of a transmissible lethal disease and an epidemic of meaning or signification." She called out the "chaotic assemblage of understandings of AIDS," all of which are attempts at "making sense" of it.[2] By now it is practically axiomatic that AIDS is a social construct in which meaning is constantly produced and reproduced. Each poster in this collection creates its own world of signification.

In some cases, historical documents reveal a great deal about who produced these posters and for whom. In others, little is known about the design or production process, and one must speculate on the makers' intentions. Designers assumed various roles in this process: some as professionals hired by national or local governmental entities, some as sympathetic collaborators with social and cultural organizations, and still others as personally engaged activists.

Whatever the designer's role, one of their primary tasks, whether working in posters or another medium, is to *translate*. This translation process is composed of two different tasks, which together attempt to communicate the author's intended message to a particular audience. The "author" here could be a public health organization, a government agency, an activist group, or the graphic designer. The audience is equally variable, such as all the residents of a city or country, gay men, or pregnant women. This represents the group the author believes require instruction or persuasion.

The designer's first task is intellectual: to understand the contexts, vocabularies, desires, and concerns of the author and the audience. What are the author's goals, immediate and long-term? What message might achieve those goals? What is the audience's current knowledge about, perception of, or resistance to that message? How, and in what terms, could these ideas be appropriately understood?

The second task is material: to transform those ideas into visual form. In graphic design—and specifically in print media—communicative intentions are made visible through unique compositions of typography, photography, drawing, and color, among other formal attributes. The end result is the designer's interpretation of the author's messaging through the imagined lens of the audience. Graphic design understood through the lens of the recipient acknowledges the designer's position between author and audience. The graphic designer is part of a political dynamic in which all three stakeholders—author, audience, and designer—are asked to negotiate the meanings under discussion and their appropriate forms of representation.

The power dynamics among authors, designers, and audiences of public health messaging in general, and with AIDS in particular, may be diverse, but they are always unbalanced. Interpretations and efficacy may vary, but a poster is not a conversation even if it intends to spark one. The poster itself cannot receive the viewer's response, although many of these posters provoked both outrage and solidarity. The authoring organization's perception of its audiences—in particular, their agency to respond positively, negatively, or at all—is an integral consideration of the design translation

itself. By what authority could an audience heed the commands of a poster? What tactic would persuade an audience to act differently or change a behavior? By what sense of common cause could an audience be compelled to trust the authoring organization as an ally in a mutual struggle? Acknowledging the audience's power to respond becomes material for the designer to visualize in the poster. In this way, posters name new subjects to reach as they also define new subjectivities around what health means to various communities.

During the late twentieth century, the world of graphic design was rapidly adopting new methods, tools, and techniques. The proliferation of computers, design software, and digital techniques transformed the worlds of images, typography, and printed media. This is to say nothing of the broader social and visual impact of the Internet. These transformations can be seen in new aesthetic dimensions made palatable by the digital realm of visual consumption and in the increasingly frenetic pace at which designers worked. With digital tools, a designer could preview a concept far more quickly and inexpensively. With the client's approval or the designer's own self-critique, the final output could then be quickly reproduced. This newfound expediency collided with the urgency of the AIDS epidemic at a critical time in the cultural evolution of graphic design. Just as many designers were questioning their future and their role in society, the AIDS epidemic gave them a social project to address.

AIDS activists of the 1980s rightly insisted that the AIDS crisis was a political crisis. From the first time the disease that would become known as AIDS was reported (1981),[3] the disease has laid bare a complex set of structural inequalities that were always about relationships among sexual practice and desire, racial segregation, and the transformations in the political economy of the late twentieth century. Despite initial reports that AIDS was a new disease that affected "otherwise healthy (white) homosexual men," AIDS was likely endemic in U.S. cities throughout the 1970s. However, because the illnesses produced by AIDS occurred among populations whose ill health was rarely recognized—poor people, people of color, intravenous drug users—AIDS, as a syndrome, was not considered notable by medical practitioners or journalists in marginalized communities.[4] The constellation of diseases produced by AIDS was further obscured and intensified by other concurrent politically tinged health crises: the war on drugs, the "end of welfare as we know it," and the skyrocketing rate of incarceration.[5] These syndemics, what public health experts define as a "set of linked health problems involving two or more afflictions," further expanded the disproportionate impact HIV/AIDS had and continues to have on disenfranchised communities in general and Black communities in particular.[6]

Gay men—consistently understood to be white, unless otherwise explicitly noted—were tied to AIDS from the start. They were quickly

"Only Gay Men Get AIDS. Only Gay Men
and Haitians Get AIDS. [...] When Are You
Going to Get It?" n.d.
Atlanta, Georgia, U.S.A.
Creator: AID Atlanta
43 x 56 cm
AP2774

"ONLY GAY MEN GET AIDS."
"ONLY GAY MEN AND HAITIANS GET AIDS."
"ONLY GAY MEN, HAITIANS, DRUG USERS AND BLOOD RECIPIENTS GET AIDS."
"ONLY GAY MEN, HAITIANS, DRUG USERS, BLOOD RECIPIENTS, BISEXUAL MEN, HETEROSEXUAL WOMEN, PROSTITUTES AND HETEROSEXUAL MEN GET AIDS."
"ONLY GAY MEN, HAITIANS, DRUG USERS, BLOOD RECIPIENTS, BISEXUAL MEN, HETEROSEXUAL WOMEN, PROSTITUTES, HETEROSEXUAL MEN, UNSUSPECTING WIVES, PREGNANT MOTHERS, BABIES AND FAMOUS ACTORS GET AIDS."
"ONLY GAY MEN, HAITIANS, DRUG USERS, BLOOD RECIPIENTS, BISEXUAL MEN, HETEROSEXUAL WOMEN, PROSTITUTES, HETEROSEXUAL MEN, UNSUSPECTING WIVES, PREGNANT MOTHERS, BABIES, FAMOUS ACTORS, FAMOUS ACTRESSES, REPUBLICANS AND DEMOCRATS GET AIDS."
"ONLY GAY MEN, HAITIANS, DRUG USERS, BLOOD RECIPIENTS, BISEXUAL MEN, HETEROSEXUAL WOMEN, PROSTITUTES, HETEROSEXUAL MEN, UNSUSPECTING WIVES, PREGNANT MOTHERS, BABIES, FAMOUS ACTORS, FAMOUS ACTRESSES, REPUBLICANS, DEMOCRATS, DOCTORS, NURSES, DENTISTS, PATIENTS, POLICE OFFICERS, CRIMINALS, FLIGHT ATTENDANTS, PILOTS, FARMERS, MANAGERS, SALESMEN, CHRISTIANS, ATHEISTS, TEACHERS, STUDENTS, SCIENTISTS, FIREMEN, DIABETICS, PROFESSIONAL ATHLETES, CALIFORNIANS, NEW YORKERS, FLORIDIANS, AMERICANS AND HUMAN BEINGS GET AIDS."

WHEN ARE YOU GOING TO GET IT?

AID
Atlanta
AIDS INFORMATION LINE 1-800-551-2728

followed by other risk groups, sometimes iden-tified as the "four Hs": homosexuals, Haitians, hemophiliacs, and heroin users.[7] Reports referred to these categories of people as *reservoirs* of the disease. This perception led to targeted calls for the containment of these identity groups.[8] Haitians, for example, could not donate blood in the United States until 1990. Gay men were banned from giving blood until 2015, when the law changed to allow them to donate only if they hadn't had sex with a man in the last twelve months.[9] The rhetoric that focused on particular identities perversely enabled people who did *not* identify with any of those catego-ries to ignore AIDS and potentially embrace a false sense of security. Assigning false blame to particular groups for the spread of AIDS also added fuel to homophobic and racist attacks on various communities.

Refuting this concept that only certain kinds of people are "going to get it," a poster, made by AID Atlanta (Atlanta is the home of the Centers for Disease Control), likely in the late 1980s, names a growing list of "risk groups." The poster visually conveys the idea that the list of identities perceived to be at risk had expanded from "gay men" all the way to "...human beings."

The unknown designer of this poster made decisive attempts to visually emphasize its message of a mounting death toll. The centered block of text surrounded by white space creates a form emblematic of a tombstone. Even the typeface is linked to naming the dead. Designed

by German typographer Hermann Zapf in the 1950s, the typeface, named *Optima,* was inspired by letterforms on tombs in Florence's Basilica of Santa Croce. It is the same typeface that lists the names of the dead on the Vietnam Veterans Memorial in Washington, D.C.

Posters such as this one underscore how activists, artists, and service providers across the United States resisted the focus on risk groups. In doing so, they constantly reframed AIDS prevention, treatment, awareness, and what it might look like to end AIDS. By the mid-1980s, AIDS workers managed to change the terms of the conversation by shifting focus from identity to behavior. The effect of this insistence influenced the messaging of most AIDS posters produced after the mid-1980s. In these posters, one can read a litany of commands to change behavior: wear a condom, clean your needles, don't have sex, fight discrimination, do some-thing, do something differently, or stop doing something altogether. By the 1990s, activists

began to call out the structural causes of AIDS—government neglect, racism, lack of universal health care—rather than suggesting individual behavior change would be sufficient. The evolu-tion of those messages is revealed in this collec-tion of posters.[10]

Zooming out to see the historical evolutions in this collection suggests that, in the United States, activists and community members deserve much of the credit for exposing the power of posters to fight AIDS. While posters made by various governmental and non-gov-ernmental public health entities have a long history (some of which is addressed in Donald Albrecht's essay herein), it appears that most of the earliest posters in this collection were produced by community-based AIDS service organizations such as GMHC (Gay Men's Health Crisis in New York) and AID Atlanta, pro-test groups such as ACT UP, political groups like the Silence = Death Collective, and activist art collectives like Gran Fury. These posters, both

"Treat People with AIDS"
(translated from French), n.d.
Series: *Uganda School Health Kit
on AIDS Control*
Kampala, Uganda
Creator: Uganda Ministry of Health,
AIDS Control Programme
60 x 42 cm
AP3411

"Stop!! Think, Say No....", n.d.
Lagos, Nigeria
Creator: Nigeria Federal Ministry of
Health, Family Planning Unit
59 x 40 cm
AP3536

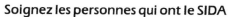
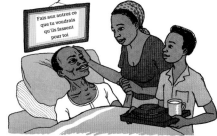

in terms of the communities they named and the kinds of demands they made, became potential sources of inspiration for larger governmental agencies that followed with national campaigns in the late 1980s and early 1990s. While we cannot substantiate this claim in other parts of the world, we can find some roots for AIDS education posters in campaigns for birth control and family planning in the global South produced in the second half of the twentieth century, as well as those calling for an end to sterilization abuse of women of color.

Acts of Interpretation

Those viewing this collection are not seeing the posters in their original contexts. The archive provides a different vantage point—one that reveals longer time lines and contexts for materials related to AIDS. The goals of this essay are twofold: to provide tools for interpreting and understanding AIDS posters; and to create context for reflection on AIDS posters, whether in this book or elsewhere. This essay integrates approaches based in graphic design and history. Graphic design's interpretive method relies on visual critique, asking questions of the formal qualities of the poster: How are photography and illustration used at turns to reify, abstract, humanize, anonymize, or to create visual or

conceptual metaphors? How do the posters connect to or refute cultural influences in the field of graphic design during the 1980s and 1990s? How does the typography carry its own connotations, unify or contrast linguistic meanings, or expand the message across global and local vocabularies?

The historical perspective focuses on the temporal, spatial, and political. What was the contemporaneous arrangement of social relationships between the publishers of the posters and their intended audiences? Is the purpose of the poster an international public health campaign, or is it created for a municipal organization aimed at influencing a social body within a more focused and local area? Is the message a voice from within that community, as in the works of ACT UP's Outreach Committee or Gran Fury?

Donald Albrecht, curator of the exhibition that accompanies this book, has selected a tiny fraction of the 8,000 posters and imagined themes from correcting misinformation to urging compassion for people with AIDS (though no doubt hundreds more exist) that frame how the posters'

visual and verbal messages function at social, political, sexual, and historical levels. This analysis suggests that the intentions of the authoring organizations that produced these posters, the designers, and their intended audiences were entangled in contexts continuously spanning the regional and global, the historical and contemporary, the aspirational and ideological.

As one of the largest collections of AIDS posters ever assembled, this will certainly be a source for future research and scholarship. As viewers practice their own interpretations, they might ask, what is the message or argument? What power does this poster, or its author, assert to make that argument? How is that argument visually or verbally signified? What new subject positions does the poster produce? Don't stop there. Consider what is *not* there and why. What questions, actions, or behaviors is the poster trying to ignore or refuse? Does it ignore certain realities in hopes of constructing the present in certain ways? How does the poster make the viewer feel?"[11]

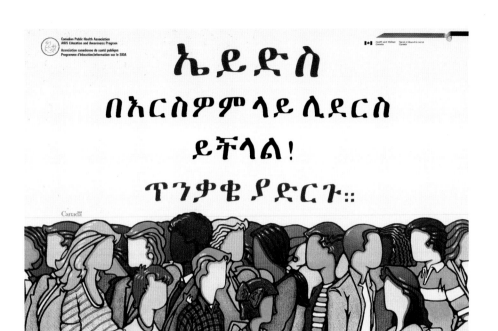

"AIDS Can Happen to You! Protect Yourself!" (translated from Amharic), n.d.
Series: *AIDS Can Happen to You!*
Canada
Creator: Canadian Public Health Association, AIDS Education and Awareness Program
42 x 56 cm
AP2279

The State Knows What's Best for Its Heterosexual Citizens

As early as 1983, it was clear that AIDS was becoming a worldwide problem. At different speeds and with different foci, countries on every continent began to create state-driven campaigns that either raised awareness about HIV/AIDS or suggested ways to thwart its spread. In every case, the local history and context shaped the visual and verbal cues that appeared on a poster. The aspirational ideals of how each country hoped to represent itself and its people did as well. This section of the essay features posters from three countries: Uganda, Nigeria, and Canada. Each poster focuses on a different kind of AIDS prevention and delivers moral instruction via verbal and visual means.

A Ugandan poster, translated from French as "Treat People with AIDS," serves to instruct women in proper behavior regarding the care of sick male relatives and the domestic work that women can perform to potentially protect themselves and their families. Illustrations are used as instructions. The poster defines gender roles of women tending to men while providing indexical information on specific tasks to reduce the spread of infection: wash hands, bandage cuts, keep the laundry clean, and do not share razors, needles, or even toothbrushes. These are domestic activities that focus on family care with no mention of sex. In contrast, a Nigerian poster addresses sexual activity by commanding abstinence: "Stop!! Think, Say No...." The illustration of a man and woman holding hands makes clear this is aimed at heterosexual relationships. The rationale for abstinence leads with unwanted pregnancy and lists AIDS last as a subset of sexually transmitted diseases.

The language and imagery in both posters are delivered by what appears to be a benevolent authority. The posters convey that authority's sense of "duty" to care for, protect, and act in ways that safeguard the nation and its citizens—as long as people maintain normative gender and sexual roles. The necessity of producing public health messages for Uganda and Nigeria, both majority Black, post-colonial countries on the African continent, was made ever more urgent as the United States and countries in Western Europe identified nations of the African diaspora, including then Zaire (now the Democratic Republic of Congo) and Haiti, as the first locations where AIDS appeared in humans. U.S. and European health and development officials and scientists regularly identified countries in central and southern Africa as poor, lacking in public health infrastructures, and not developed to explain the global AIDS pandemic. In her essay "From Nation to Family: Containing African AIDS," Cindy Patton explains that "Whatever the overt concerns of international health workers for containing AIDS in (within?) the continent, their construal of 'Africa' as the margin of economic/cultural 'development' and as the 'heart' of the AIDS epidemic helps to stabilize a Euro-America adrift in a postmodern condition of lost metanarratives and occluded origins."[12] For Patton, this postmodern condition was deeply colonial. It always named Africa as a "dark" place where AIDS began, not as a continent of more than fifty countries struggling to survive and thrive in a post-colonial and structurally unequal world.

The Canadian Public Health Association's AIDS Education and Awareness Program produced the third poster in this grouping as part of a set of twelve posters designed to reach the largest ethnic immigrant groups in Canada in the 1990s. Published in Amharic, the national language of Ethiopia, as well

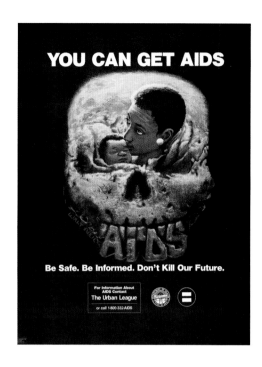

"You Can Get AIDS," 1988
Ohio, U.S.A.
Creator: Ohio Department of Health
36 x 28 cm
AP1383

as eleven other languages (English, Chinese, Hindi, Spanish, Haitian Creole, Arabic, French, Vietnamese, Khmer, Somali, and Persian), each poster contained an identical image and message. "AIDS Can Happen to You! Protect Yourself!" is emblazoned over an illustration of a faceless crowd. Ages and ethnicities (represented by different skin tones and hair colors and textures) are abstracted and clearly diverse, but the clothes are all the same. They show no evidence of sexuality, except for a blonde woman prominently cradling her own pregnant form to remind the viewer of the intergenerational and presumably heterosexual risks at stake. The posters express no substantive command beyond "protect yourself!" The federal mark of Canada (with maple leaf) is carefully positioned just above the head of the pregnant blonde woman, ensuring our gaze will not miss her. Everyone is vulnerable, even the unborn.

As a set, the posters reflect how Canada imagines itself as a pluralistic nation of immigrants, while deftly ignoring its settler-colonial past and present. While the posters were translated into twelve languages, no poster was made in Anishinaabe, a language of the First Nation people of Ottawa, seat of Canada's national government. This omission amounts to ignoring the prevalence of AIDS among First Nations people and on Native lands.

The three posters portray, to varying degrees, a sense of distance between the publishing organizations and their audiences.

Whether they convey a sense of collective responsibility or a more pointed message that "you are responsible," the audience is perceived to be ignorant of the proper procedures of health and protection. These audiences don't grasp the risks or the appropriate measures of prevention; they must be instructed. The posters also reveal deeply held national conceptions of the epidemic. Each nation names and defines how its ideal(ized) citizens should act, and how it plans to address AIDS within its borders.

Scaring You Straight

Back in the United States, local entities, such as state-level public health departments and municipal AIDS service organizations, made posters that targeted more specific communities, and regularly employed the language of fear in materials meant to control AIDS. While taking many forms, the message was often arresting: this disease will kill you; it will kill your family; it will harm your unborn children. The visual metaphors used include bodies in the morgue, tombstones, skulls, and a whole gallery of monstrous fictional characters, some wielding needles, and others donning crutches or bandages.

These posters use fear. They seek to make people understand how they *should live*. In many cases, however, no particular behavior change is named. The "scare you straight" approach imagines a person's lifestyle is a choice they can change at will. Simply getting the message will be enough to produce "improvement."

One example, a poster created by the Ohio Department of Health with the Urban League, targeted African-American mothers for AIDS awareness and prevention. The poster's text, however, did not make evident what it wanted them to "be informed" about or "be safe" from. Instead the image of a mother comforting her child within a skull haunts the viewer, hoping that the woman will somehow protect both herself and her baby. What we cannot see in this 1988 poster is that Ohio required mandatory reporting, by name, of people diagnosed with AIDS. Thus, when the poster was produced, the state of Ohio already had a list, by name, of all 200 Ohioans who had been diagnosed with the disease. While we do not know which communities were the intended audience for this poster, its signification begs some questions: What was the relationship between state surveillance and state-sponsored awareness campaigns? In particular, how effective could state campaigns have been in preventing the spread of HIV if the state was actively involved in health-related surveillance? Since the state was "informed" of who was infected, what information did the viewers

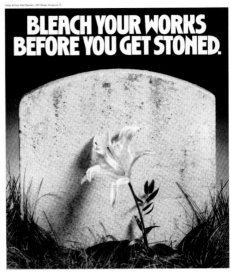

"Bleach Your Works before You Get Stoned," before 1989
Series: *Don't Let This AIDS Message Be in Vein*
Providence, Rhode Island, U.S.A.
Creator: Rhode Island AIDS Project
Designer and writer: Peter Spameni
66 x 46 cm
AP5145

"Flexible Life Insurance," n.d.
Auckland, New Zealand
Creator: New Zealand AIDS Foundation
85 x 60 cm
AP3112

of this poster gain? Was safety something the Black mother pictured in the poster could enact for herself, or was the state of Ohio's intervention required to change the mother's behavior? This poster offered no solutions or options of what to do to stay alive, while others perpetuated the idea that women were vectors for AIDS and regularly put their children at risk. By 2017, Black women were more likely to contract HIV than any other group of women in the state of Ohio by an order of magnitude.[13]

Harm Reduction

While some populations were commanded to be scared to death about AIDS, others were provided with the visual and verbal language of harm reduction. That is, the idea that it is possible to lessen the likelihood of spreading HIV by changing the way intravenous drugs are used. Sparked by activists and service providers working with IV drug users, harm reduction recognizes that people need not stop using drugs (in contrast, think of Nancy Reagan's call to "Just Say No" in the 1980s) to lower their risk of contracting HIV. Instead, those building a case

for harm reduction argue people should have access to clean needles through either needle exchange or easily accessible mechanisms to clean their "works." San Francisco's Prevention Point, for example, produced a series of posters with the tagline "Just Say Know," demonstrating the turn from messages persuading viewers to abstain from "high-risk" activities to instead doing them more safely. The series included the bold tagline in conjunction with images of both needles and condoms.

Another series of posters, published by the AIDS Council of New South Wales in the late 1980s, focused on "Household Tips for Drug Users" and "Safe Sex Made Simple." They used a comic book approach of multiple characters in short, sequential narratives. Cartoonist Kaz Cooke's well-known character "Hermione, the Modern Girl" instructs a sunglasses-wearing dude wearing a shirt that reads, "I [heart] Condoms & Speed" that he should bleach his needle or get a new, free one. In a dark turn, he proposes drinking the bleach.

Combining the language of harm reduction with a dose of fear, a 1980s poster published

by the Rhode Island AIDS project was copywritten and designed by Peter Spameni—at the time a recent graduate of the Rhode Island School of Design. The poster reads, "Bleach Your Works before You Get Stoned." The typography is bold, reversed out of a black-and-white photograph of a lily growing from the earth in front of a blank headstone. The image and typographic treatment seem more redolent of a rock album cover than a public health message. The metaphoric language is nuanced enough to wink at intravenous drug users in its audience by speaking their slang. In this landscape, drug users are not idiotic villains. Instead, they are sophisticated, culturally savvy consumers. In a broader cultural context, Everett True, definitive author of the history of the grunge rock band Nirvana, claims that the band named their debut album "Bleach" (1989) after singer-songwriter Kurt Cobain saw this poster while he was on tour in San Francisco.[14] This open exchange of cultural ideas between a public health poster and a rock band—one on the verge of transforming the international music scene, including redefining public perceptions of heroin use—demonstrates just how attuned this young poster designer was to his intended audience.

A more visually and verbally aggressive example of the harm reduction approach can be seen in the 1996 poster by the San Francisco AIDS Foundation promoting their needle exchange program, which reads, "Death Is Not an Option." The graphic forms are undeniably representative of the time: tightly cropped, tortured, and textured letter forms bleed into the crumpled paper surface. Splatters and smears of ink evince an act of craft and labor—a constructed graphic object, not a clean, efficient, digital work. No needles are shown. Instead, the aesthetic presentation carries the context. Fine print didactic text appears below the tagline and reads, "You Know What's Going On. You Can Do Whatever You Want. You Can Choose to Live." Given its design aesthetic, this poster asks viewers to understand the motifs of avant-garde advertising. It would be at home with contemporaneous ads for designer blue jeans or sneakers.

Advertising AIDS

At the same time that harm reduction strategies were making certain kinds of AIDS prevention visible, a strand of social advertising amplified the argument that *everyone* is at risk of contracting AIDS. *Everyone* in these representations usually means white heterosexual people, akin to the universalist claim that AIDS does not discriminate.

The language of universal risk, for example, runs as the tagline at the bottom of a New Zealand condom ad: "Every 10 Minutes Someone, Somewhere, Dies of AIDS. Before You're Going to Have Sex, Stop and Think: Are

You Covered?" This text requires tapping into a combination of a sense of sameness and consumption. The unnamed individuals or communities targeted by this poster and others like it are often assumed to be visually and intellectually sophisticated. To convince them, the designer must pique their self-interest and tap into their economic aspirations as consumers. This is advertising working toward the production of lifestyle types, creating norms and choices.

What posters like this one miss is that despite universal claims that AIDS affects everybody, it does not affect everybody in the same ways, for the same reasons, or at the same magnitude. The "protect yourself" movement imagined equity in access to AIDS prevention. The call to individual responsiblity did not match the reality of social, economic, or health conditions for the people most directly affected by AIDS. These posters and their phrasing have a way of further denying the reality that AIDS is actually fueled by inequality and that people are able to make choices free of political, economic, and social constraints.

Queer (White Male) Design

From the first reported cases of the disease that would later be named AIDS in the United States, AIDS has been associated with gay men and, later, with men who have sex with men (MSM). The default assumption of what "gay" means has almost always been based on a particular white masculine model. This was true even as

gay activists and service providers created the idea of *safe sex*, later renamed *safer sex*, and white gay male designers put it into visual form. The detailing of safer sex was a cantankerous process, but, at its core, it was meant to persuade gay men to fundamentally transform their sexual behavior. This transition toward persuasively signifying changes in sexual practice took many forms, including the deeply erotic. The concept of safer sex, including its rituals, accessories, and a new vocabulary, became a "lifestyle" or "product" to be sold, even though the intended audiences were not identical or even necessarily connected. Lifestyle images became normative, shaping new subjectivities of how to live, even as they attempted to reach a variety of social groups.

From 1988 to 1990, the San Francisco AIDS Foundation (SFAF), one of the first and largest AIDS service organizations in the United States, designed a series of posters to address the safer sex messaging and tested them on different racial and ethnic gay communities in the city. In each poster, the imagery explicitly connects a short tagline to condom use within a modernist logic of semiotics: the image and language simultaneously contextualize each other to make meaning from the whole.

One such poster, "Dress for the Occasion," features a seated nude white man with an erect penis sheathed in a condom. The tagline implies an affluent class status: the man's birthday suit subbing for a tuxedo or fashion-forward suit and tie. Designed to be displayed in bars, the poster

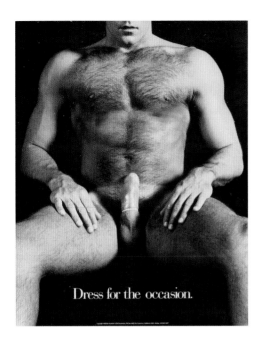

Dress for the occasion.

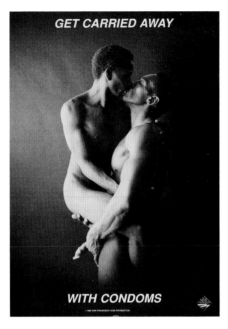

GET CARRIED AWAY

WITH CONDOMS

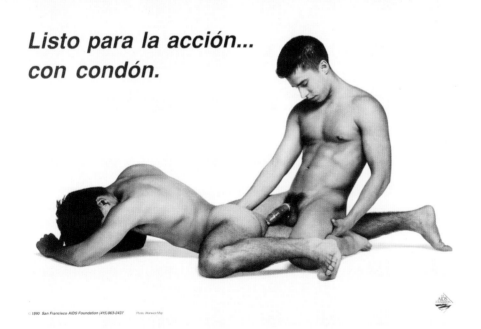

Listo para la acción... con condón.

© 1990 San Francisco AIDS Foundation (415) 863-2437   Photo: Warwick May

"Dress for the Occasion," 1988
San Francisco, California, U.S.A.
Creator: San Francisco AIDS Foundation
50 x 39 cm
AP349

"Get Carried Away with Condoms," 1990
San Francisco, California, U.S.A.
Creator: San Francisco AIDS Foundation
52 x 36 cm
AP350

"Ready for Action...with a Condom"
(translated from Spanish), 1990
San Francisco, California, U.S.A.
Creator: San Francisco AIDS Foundation
Designer: Warwick May
36 x 52 cm
AP352

campaign seems to have targeted the gay community in San Francisco. While only the bottom of the man's face is in the frame, his traditionally masculine white body was intended to have universal appeal as a man ready for action.

In contrast to "Dress for the Occasion," "Get Carried Away with Condoms" features a Black male couple kissing and embracing one another and showing one man holding his partner off the ground, his partner's legs wrapped around his torso. They are preparing to have "safer sex"— with a condom. The picture is both erotic and intimate, deeply committed to showing Black love. Accompanying brochures on topics such as cleaning needles further called attention to Black men's multiple risks. The Get Carried Away campaign was one of two that targeted specific racial or ethnic groups of gay men. The other was for Latinos, "Listo para la acción con condón" ("Ready for Action with a Condom"). It appeared in Spanish-speaking bars catering to gay Latinos.

Archival materials held at the University of California at San Francisco AIDS History Project indicate significant controversy around both the design process and distribution of these

"Beyond Big Dicked Bottoms," 1998
Series: *Q Action*
San Francisco, California, U.S.A.
Creator: Stop AIDS Project
Designer: Peter Koblish
49 x 26 cm
AP2756

"Future Forward," 1997
Series: *Q Action*
San Francisco, California, U.S.A.
Creator: Stop AIDS Project
Designer: Martin Venezky
56 x 26 cm
AP2751

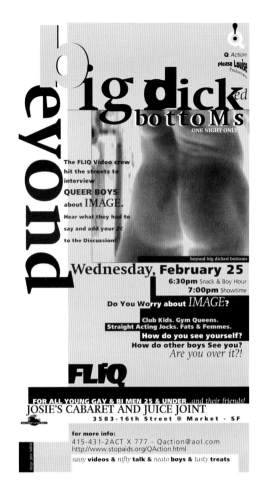

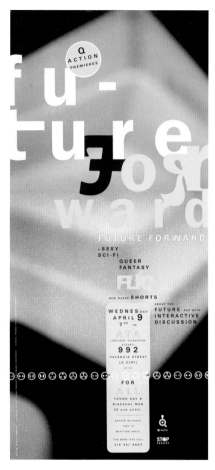

materials in that city. In part, the dispute was over how gay men of color should be represented in materials made by a majority-white organization and intended for audiences made up of men of color. In essence, in what ways could race, in general, and black- and brown-ness, in particular, be depicted so that men could identify with the images and commit to behavior change? How would the histories of racism, particularly those that brutalized supposedly "overly sexual" men of color, be accounted for? Also part of the kerfuffle was the U.S. government's censorship of materials deemed to be "promoting homosexuality," or what some have termed the "no promohomo," law supported by Republican Senator Jesse Helms of North Carolina.[15] In this case, a local board of reviewers revealed a double standard by authorizing a print run of the poster for Black men, but refusing to fund the campaign for Latino gay men because it was too sexually explicit. To mass produce the Latino poster, SFAF had to allocate privately raised money. No state resources were used in safer sex campaigns for this targeted group because community review board evaluators argued that the materials presented images and arguments that violated community standards.[16]

Near the end of the twentieth century, posters produced by and for AIDS activist groups in San Francisco shifted to name queer communities as necessary targets. Following a similar transition in political organizing (Queer Nation began its direct-action work in 1990 in New York City), posters from STOP AIDS San Francisco[17] reclaimed the hostile epithet to suggest that fighting AIDS required reaching queer men who were often rejected by overtly masculine gay norms. "Fats and Femmes," for example, were told to disavow their own mistreatment and embrace who they were.

Transformations in gay/queer organizing ran parallel to radical changes in the field of graphic design, where a clash of ideologies was fueled by broader cultural and aesthetic debates on the problematic nature of universal claims prevalent in modernist design. This evolution from gay to queer was analogous to the shift from the universally applicable, demographically targeted communication logics of modernism to the postmodern. Graphic designers translated postmodernist (and post-structuralist) challenges to the grand narratives and stable aesthetic sensibilities of modernism. The innovators of this approach collided disparate visual materials—vernacular typographic forms, found images, low-resolution reproduction techniques, raucous and sometimes jarring combinations and scales of letterforms, perversions of spelling and syntax—in ways that similarly challenged prevailing semantic and aesthetic norms. This was not a clever (albeit confusing) presentation of a message, but rather a challenge to the *possibility* of conveying a single, coherent message.

As discursive and aesthetic possibilities proliferated through the use of digital image-making tools, the posters accentuated the multiplicity of sexual identities and expressions. Posters, for example, produced for the Q Action[18] film series by the STOP AIDS Project, demonstrate what would have been an emergent aesthetic sensibility of postmodernist design. The influence of San Francisco-based *Emigre* magazine, with its designers who were early adopters of Macintosh computers for layout design, can also be seen in many of these posters.[19] Promoting the screening of the Q Action documentary *Beyond Big Dicked Bottoms*, a poster designed by Peter Koblish asks, "Do you worry about image?" The playful but chaotic mix of letterforms, scale, inverted photography, and use of color for drawing out a shifting grid structure are emblematic of the postmodernist movement. While the photograph is distorted and anonymous, it is still a clearly identifiable reference to the male anatomy.

Martin Venezky, another San Francisco graphic designer, created posters and ephemera for Q Action from 1996 to 2000. This was shortly after his graduate education at the Cranbrook Academy of Art, where he studied with Katherine McCoy, one of the progenitors of postmodern and post-structuralist thinking in graphic design.[20] Venezky's 1998 poster for Q Action's "Future Forward" event extends the burgeoning postmodernist concepts of Koblish's poster even further. Mixed scales

and types of letterforms merge with snippets of blurred, out-of-focus, photos and a series of difficult-to-interpret icons. Together they de-stabilize any clear subject-object relationships and create a floating set of referents. Is this an ad for a technology conference, a consumer product, or a targeted film series for a specific community? Context, in this poster, is everything. Meaning is fleeting; representation may be impossible.

The posters featured from the Q Action series were also created after the advent of protease inhibitors and suggest that gay and bisexual men would be at the forefront of stopping AIDS. Community members have the knowledge and ability to make one another healthy. In some ways, the aesthetic dimensions of these posters *are* the message. Similar graphic languages would be recognizable from flyers and handbills promoting DJs and events at gay male clubs in the city. In this aesthetic transfer from literary theory to promoting club life and film series on serious questions facing the gay community, design translates hyper-contextualized visual ideas separately from the posters' verbal content.

Protest Posters: End AIDS, End White Heteropatriarchal Capitalism

By the late 1980s and early 1990s, dramatic changes in image production were made possible through digital technologies. Yet, along with them came a fracturing of meanings and audiences. As the culture wars of the 1980s rambled into this new *becoming-digital* culture,

various social and interest groups produced media for their own purposes of communication and protest. These HIV/AIDS posters protested major institutions—the government, the church, various health organizations—and called out powerful individuals by name, such as former President Ronald Reagan, Republican Senator Jesse Helms, New York's Cardinal John O'Connor, and Dr. Anthony S.Fauci of the National Institute of Allergy and Infectious Diseases. The posters even featured fictional personalities, such as the Marlboro Man, as the face of corporate interests that supported homophobic and "AIDS-phobic" politicians and "legislative bigotry."

Gran Fury, the artist-activist collective that grew out of ACT UP, produced notoriously provocative images such as the bloody handprint in "The Government Has Blood on Its Hands" and the "Kissing Doesn't Kill" public art project. A 1994 poster by *Colors* magazine (published by Benetton under the editorial direction of Tibor Kalman and Olivero Toscani) famously featured a supposedly AIDS-stricken Ronald Reagan, using a photo that was manipulated so that he appeared to have Kaposi's sarcoma lesions all over his face. Such image manipulations were initially criticized for using "real" photographs to promote "unreal" narratives. Kalman's response was that "photography is not objective; it never has been objective."[21] This discourse was unfolding at the same time that digital tools for easily manipulating photographic

AIDS: GOVERNMENT NEGLECT PUBLIC INDIFFERENCE

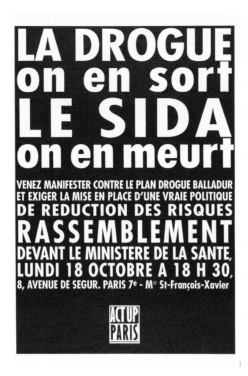

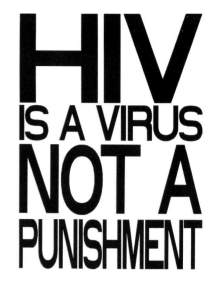

"AIDS: Government Neglect,
Public Indifference," n.d.
New York, New York, U.S.A.
Creator: ACT UP
77 x 51 cm
AP1175

"Drugs One Can Quit. AIDS Kills You"
(translated from French), 1993
Paris, France
Creator: ACT UP Paris
60 x 40 cm
AP6602

"HIV Is a Virus, Not a Punishment," 1994
Series: High School
Hamilton, Ontario, Canada
Creator: Hamilton AIDS Network for
Dialogue and Support
43 x 28 cm
AP2127

images—perhaps, most prominently, Adobe Photoshop®—were becoming more accessible and commonly used by designers.

Readers of the Benetton magazine have rightly criticized the corporation for inserting AIDS into its global advertising campaign. Prior to the founding of *Colors* magazine, co-editor and photographer Oliver Toscani worked on several Benetton ad campaigns that included provocative imagery with a Benetton logo as the only tagline. While these criticisms are valid, for our purposes of interpretation, it should be noted that in examples like the Reagan poster, the language of advertising is applied in a way distinct from that seen in condom ads referenced earlier in this essay. This manipulated image was not directly selling products. Nor was it selling new subjectivities in the form of new lifestyles that include safer or healthier living. Instead, the designers hoped to galvanize global audiences to see how the U.S. government and president were responsible for AIDS looking the way it did in 1994. It was political art.

A sense of urgency is palpable in protest posters with bold, sometimes crude, typographic compositions that occasionally veer toward *undesign.* The total absence of photographs or other visual representations of people or objects is also worth noting. The immediacy made manifest in these posters focuses on language, while the visual forms are reminiscent of block-printed broadsides or early tools of desktop publishing—both technologies that have radically democratized the production of graphic artifacts. Posters such as one that announces "AIDS: Government Neglect, Public Indifference" echo the "I Am a Man" posters carried in protests after the 1968 assassination of Dr. Martin Luther King, Jr.[22] In that movement, declarations of basic personhood carried powerful significance.

Another instance of this bold typographic strategy is a series of posters published by the Hamilton AIDS Network in Canada, one of the first nations where calls to eliminate laws making HIV transmission a crime took root. "HIV Is a

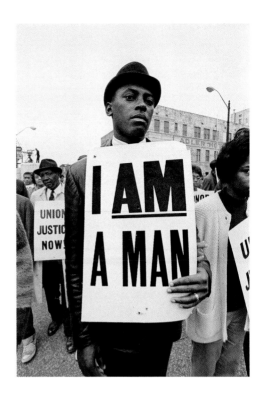

"I Am a Man Strike, Memphis, Tennessee,"
1968
Photo: Bob Adelman

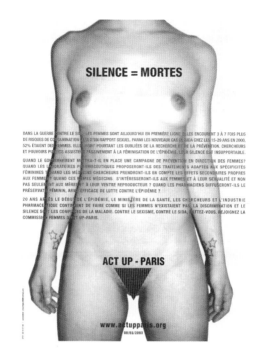

"Silence = Death" (translated from French),
2003
Paris, France
Creator: ACT UP Paris
70 x 50 cm
AP6493

Virus, Not a Punishment" reads one of the posters from the series. The black words are bold and stark against the white background, and they grab viewers' attention by a subtle but visually jarring move: a sans serif example of what's called a reverse-contrast letterform. Traditionally, Latin characters have thicker vertical strokes than their horizontal strokes—a quality these forms developed in over 2,000 years of use from stone-carving through calligraphy to letterpress. In the early nineteenth century, such eccentric reverse-contrast typefaces were used on posters to deliberately attract attention—"a dirty trick," according to designer Peter Bil'ak, "to create freakish letterforms that stood out in the increasingly saturated world of commercial messages."[23] We can't be sure if the designer of this poster was intentionally revisiting this maneuver from typographic history to create a similar attention-grabbing "trick." Regardless, this would have been an odd (or novel) typographic decision, surely intended to cut through the commercial visual clutter of Canadian streetscapes in the 1990s.

In a similar way, pithy and memorable statements such as ACT UP's "Silence = Death" carried complex ideas in a compact linguistic package.[24] Posters with this statement (first in English, then in many languages) appeared with an upward-pointing pink triangle. Badges with a downward-pointing pink triangle had been used in Nazi concentration camps in the 1930s and 1940s to mark prisoners by their sexual orientations or identities (homosexual men, bisexual men, and transgender women). This symbol was reclaimed by the LGBTQ community in the 1970s—adjusted to an upward-pointing pink triangle—to positively re-appropriate its use in protests against homophobia. The pink triangle situates the statement "Silence = Death" within a protest movement around homophobia, sexuality, and AIDS, while the statement itself demonstrates how simple language can carry complex ideas into different territories of AIDS "signification."

Later versions of this messaging brought direct contact with photographic imagery. In a French ACT UP poster from 2003, for example, the downward-pointing triangle is carefully positioned over a woman's genitals to allow public posting, while three full paragraphs of pink typography are fully overprinted on a black-and-white photo. Digital design tools and experiences in early web design both would have made it easier for designers to "see" text blocks (body copy) overlaying images, and thus guaranteeing legibility. What we observe is the language developing its signification first in conjunction with the symbol (pink triangle), then on its own, then in various configurations with other images. This process produces added meaning: men are not the only ones who matter when we think about or act against AIDS.

Conclusion

As the world moves into its fifth decade of the presence of AIDS, we return to where we began: We all live with AIDS. A 2018 poster by Chicago-based artist Charles Ryan Long and Christopher Paul Jordan from Tacoma, Washington, refuses structural violence and racism. In detailing the inspiration and purpose of the poster, Long writes that it was meant to "mimic slave catcher" posters from the antebellum period in Boston.[25] The poster's explicit criticism of HIV criminalization and the policing of people living with AIDS (which in this case means the policing of all of us) is amplified by the choice of font and lettering that is meant to look like a warning issued to those who might have harbored enslaved people in the 1850s. What is required for these graphic artists is to build political affinities and collective conceptions of health and well-being.

"Attention!!! People Living with AIDS," 2018
Chicago, Illinois, U.S.A.
Creators and designers: Charles Ryan
Long in collaboration with Christopher
Paul Jordan
56 x 25.5 cm
AP50075

If AIDS is to end, the political, cultural, and social structures that exacerbate inequality and make people sick need to change. This is particularly hard to do because public health organizations have historically operated as institutions that normalize conceptions of health as individual decisions; yet norms can also be adapted, re-oriented, or flat-out rejected by the populations affected by these normalizing constructs.

The sense of urgency that compelled many designers to just do "something"—in collaboration with health or social organizations or as activists themselves—still persists in the world of graphic design. All forms of visual communication are affected by digital forces, one way or another. In turn, the focus returns to the human concerns of living within our fully digitized world. Graphic designers are today seen adopting various communicative strategies to convey "urgency" or "authenticity." That aim for immediacy has further mutated in the age of social media. The poster, while still a hallmark of graphic meaning-making, is no longer the primary "mode" of proximal, local, and already-contextualized communication it once was. Today, images of persuasion—and, indeed, propaganda—swirl in digital space in ways that posters never could or were intended to do. The "crisis" of signification continues for AIDS. The sense of a shared "reality" is difficult, if not impossible, to conjure, and competing significations of power and subjectivity have become further fragmented.

ATTENTION!!!

PEOPLE LIVING WITH AIDS
(BY WHICH WE MEAN EVERYONE ON THE GLOBE)

You are hereby respectfully encouraged to end all tolerance of *RACIST, SEXIST, TRANSPHOBIC, XENOPHOBIC, SEX NEGATIVE & CLASSIST* individuals, systems and governments.

they may be police
the may be a case worker
they may be your neighbor
they may be male (or using toxic masculinity)
they may be a lover or a trick
YOU MUST BE DILIGENT
Institutions have been created to
massacre, enslave, rape
and pillage the people, the lands and the worker.

But **WE ARE HERE** although they deem us,
our actions and bodies illegal and therefore cageable
they will never succeed.

For we the Black, the Brown, the undocumented,
the Female, the Non-Cis, the sex worker, the sissy, the dyke, the
faggot, the user, the poor, the poz and the neg know better.

We are HIV$_x$

Notes

1. Paula Treichler first coined the term in her essay "AIDS, Homophobia, and Biomedical Discourse: An Epidemic of Signification," in *Cultural Studies*, based on a talk at the MLA. The essay is reprinted in her critical collection *How to Have Theory in an Epidemic* (Durham, NC: Duke University Press, 1999).

2. Treichler, 32–34.

3. In New York, Los Angeles, and San Francisco.

4. See, for example, Michelle Cochrane, *When AIDS Began: San Francisco and the Making of an Epidemic* (Abingdon-on-Thames, England: Routledge, 2003).

5. While the literature on the political and social transformations of the late twentieth century is well beyond the scope of this essay, we encourage interested readers to consult Elizabeth Hinton, *From the War on Poverty to the War on Crime: The Making of Mass Incarceration in America* (Cambridge, MA: Harvard University Press, 2017); Dorothy Roberts, *Killing the Black Body: Race, Reproduction and the Meaning of Liberty* (New York: Vintage Books, 1998); Michelle Alexander, *The New Jim Crow: Mass Incarceration in the Age of Colorblindness* (New York: New Press, 2012); and Felicia Kornbluh and Gwendolyn Mink, *Ensuing Poverty: Welfare Reform in Feminist Perspective* (Philadelphia, PA: University of Pennsylvania Press, 2018).

6. For further reading on syndemics, see https://www.medicinenet.com/script/main/art.asp?articlekey=22591 (accessed March 17, 2020). For further reading on AIDS and Blackness, there is a rich and interdisciplinary literature in public health, anthropology, history, and literary studies. Two of the original and key texts continue to be Cathy Cohen, *The Boundaries of Blackness: AIDS and the Breakdown of Black Politics* (Chicago, IL: University of Chicago Press, 1999); and Evelynn Hammonds, "Race, Sex, AIDS: The Construction of 'Other,'" *Radical America* 20, no. 6 (1987): 328–40. More recent work includes Celeste Watkins-Hayes, *Remaking a Life: How Women Living with HIV/AIDS Confront Inequality* (Oakland, CA: University of California Press, 2019); Dagmawi Woubshet, *The Calendar of Loss: Race, Sexuality, and Morning in the Early Era of AIDS* (Baltimore, MD: Johns Hopkins University Press, 2015); Darius Bost, *Evidence of Being: The Black Gay Cultural Renaissance and the Politics of Violence* (Chicago, IL: University of Chicago Press, 2019); and Marlon B. Bailey and Darius Bost, eds., "The Black AIDS Epidemic," *Souls*, 21, nos. 2 and 3 (2019), the double issue features prose, poetry and art on the Black AIDS epidemic.

7. See Treichler, *How to Have Theory*, 20.

8. Paula Treichler, "AIDS, Homophobia, and Biomedical Discourse: An Epidemic of Signification," *October*, vol. 43 (Winter, 1987), 36.

9. A great deal has been written about the ban on gay men, most recently in relation to donating blood during the COVID-19 pandemic. See https://www.theguardian.com/us-news/2020/apr/18/us-blood-donation-gay-men-coronavirus (accessed April 26, 2020).

10. The historical literature on AIDS is growing. See Jennifer Brier, *Infectious Ideas: U.S. Political Reponses to the AIDS Crisis* (Chapel Hill, NC: University of North Carolina Press, 2009); Deborah Gould, *Moving Politics: Emotion and Shifting Political Horizons in the Fight Against AIDS* (Chicago, IL: University of Chicago Press, 2009); and Roger Hallas, *Reframing Bodies: AIDS, Bearing Witness, and the Queer Moving Image* (Durham, NC: Duke University Press, 2009). For a longer historiographical review see "HIV/AIDS and U.S. History," *Journal of American History* 104, no. 2 (September 1, 2017): 431–60; and Jih-Fei Cheng, Alexandra Juhasz and Nishant Shahani, co-editors, *AIDS and the Distribution of Crises* (Durham, NC: Duke University Press, forthcoming).

11. As we revised this essay, we learned of Douglas Crimp's death. A long-time member of the University of Rochester faculty, Crimp was one of the most important scholar activists writing about AIDS. His work has been foundational to what we know and feel about AIDS within the academic field and activist context, he was internationally known. Were he alive, it would be very strange for him not to appear in this book as an author. Crimp's work on AIDS emotion should be required reading for people interested in AIDS posters. See Douglas Crimp, *Melancholia and Moralism: Essays on AIDS and Queer Politics* (Cambridge, MA: MIT Press, 2002).

12. Cindy Patton, "From Nation to Family: Containing African AIDS," in Henry Abelove, et al., eds., *The Lesbian and Gay Studies Reader* (New York and London: Routledge, 1993): 127. See also Patton's Globalizing AIDS (Minneapolis, MN: University of Minnesota Press, 2002).

13. Ohio Department of Health, "HIV in Ohio," https://odh.ohio.gov/wps/wcm/connect/gov/2af5d7eb-b1e3-4df7-bbd2-9fe-6c493a8ad/Ohio+HIV+Summary+2017.pdf?MOD=AJPERES&CONVERT_TO=url&CACHEID=ROOTWORKSPACE.Z18_M1HGGIK0N0JO00QO9DDDDM3000-2af5d7eb-b1e3-4df7-bbd2-9fe6c493a8ad-mlp3cfU (accessed June 20, 2019).

14. Everett True, *Nirvana: The Biography* (Cambridge, MA: Da Capo Press, 2006), 118.

15. Robert Hunt Ferguson, "Mothers Against Jesse in Congress: Grassroots Maternalism and the Cultural Politics of the AIDS Crisis in North Carolina," *Journal of Southern History* 83, no. 1 (2017): 107–40.

16. For a fuller discussion of these campaigns and the internal struggles of the San Francisco AIDS Foundation, see Brier, *Infectious Ideas*, Chapter 2.

17. Dedicated to being a sex-positive San Francisco group, STOP AIDS was a small grassroots organization started in 1984/5 with the mission of providing gay men with the space to discuss how to end AIDS. With a focus on dialogue and sex instead of just sex, STOP AIDS sought to help gay, queer, and men who have sex with men sustain their adoption of safer sex.

18. Q meaning queer, and expressly not gay, non-normative, or radical.

19. Emigre Magazine, "Emigre Fonts," https://www.emigre.com/Magazine (accessed June 20, 2019).

20. Ethan Edwards, "Way Out West: The work of recent Cranbrook graduate Martin Venezky indicates new directions in the academy (*sic*)," *Eye Magazine* (Autumn 1993), http://www.eyemagazine.com/feature/article/way-out-west (accessed April 22, 2020).

21. Tibor Kalman, "Photography, Morality, and Benetton" (1993), in Peter Hall and Michael Bierut, eds., *Tibor Kalman: Perverse Optimist* (New York: Princeton Architectural Press, 1998).

22. Steve Estes, *I am a Man!: Race, Manhood and the Civil Rights Movement* (Chapel Hill, NC: University of North Carolina Press, 2005).

23. Peter Bil'ak, I Love Typography, "Beauty and Ugliness in Type design" (September 25, 2012), https://ilovetypography.com/2012/09/25/beauty-and-ugliness-in-type-font-design/ (accessed June 20, 2019).

24. For a stunning historical account of "Silence=Death" see Avram Finkelstein, *After Silence: A History of AIDS through Its Images* (Oakland, CA: University of California Press, 2017).

25. Brier interview with Charles Long, August 23, 2019.

Poster Portfolio

Introduction by Ian Bradley-Perrin
Curated by Donald Albrecht

Introduction

Ian Bradley-Perrin

The portfolio of approximately 150 HIV/AIDS posters includes extended captions for about two dozen of them. The people who wrote these texts include poster designers and activists, researchers and policymakers, historians, social scientists, and healthcare providers. Several are people living with HIV whose lives have been shaped by these posters. An international group of contributors was invited to choose among the more than 8,000 posters in the University of Rochester's collection and, in brief commentaries, tell stories about their choices. Responses encompassed the personal, political, professional, and aesthetic. They spanned the breadth of the posters' encounters with the world.

Some of the selections offered striking juxtapositions, none more so than two posters exploring the concept of silence: "Silence = Death" and "Silence = Sex." The first was the canonical piece of AIDS agitprop from the 1980s that was drafted into service by numerous activist groups within the AIDS movement (and since then for causes across the political spectrum). Dr. Anthony S. Fauci, involved with AIDS research from the 1980s, attested to the impact that this poster made on policymaking through the mobilization it facilitated. The poster's effectiveness was a credit to the thoughtful and intentional process of its creation, which drew on the artistic, political, and commercial experiences of the Silence = Death Collective that produced it. Nearly three decades later,

"Silence = Sex" reused the iconic design and particularly the fine print to which Jordan Arseneault has directed our attention in his text. Arseneault did this to call out the social and policy failures of HIV criminalization and its impact on interpersonal relationships through stigma as well as through impediments to HIV testing.

Other posters singled out by contributors played with advertising, including the marketers' use of fine print and branding imagery. For example, "Enjoy AZT," inspired by Coca Cola ads, was chosen by two contributors—one its creator, Avram Finkelstein, and the second, Dr. Stephen Dewhurst, a doctor and researcher who encountered it as a graduate student, and who has spent his career in search of an inexpensive HIV vaccine. Advocacy poster designers often employed fine print to convey double messages to different audiences. "AIDS Causes Blindness," for instance, relied on fine print to deliver a two-tiered message; it was selected by Dr. Joseph N. Lambert, an ophthalmologist who reflected on the dual connotations of physical and cultural blindness.

Contributors also addressed advertising posters adopting a social conscience. In his contribution, Theodore Kerr dug into the way that the United Colors of Benetton poster of David Kirby on his deathbed made the reality of AIDS visible to a massive public, while the consumer media that enabled such visibility did not tell the full story of the intimate and personal relationships the poster depicted. At the same time, Sur Rodney (Sur) considered how the use of Ronald Reagan's portrait in the company's *Colors* campaign was edited to depict him with Kaposi's sarcoma (KS) lesions. For Sur, who had witnessed Reagan's callous response to people dying of AIDS with the full visibility of KS, the *Colors* campaign took on a double life, both commercial and personal.

Numerous posters chosen by contributors took up public health policies and practices that have been enacted by governments and critiqued by advocacy organizations. As Mats Christiansen noted in his discussion of the poster "Candle March," Swedish policies in the 1990s relied on criminalization and challenged the rights of those affected. Similarly, Japan's immigration ban, which emerged in the 1990s when AIDS was already a global pandemic and treatment was increasingly effective, prompted the poster selection of Kyle Croft. Ken Monteith's analysis of the campaign featuring coffins by COCQ-SIDA (Coalition of Québec Community Organizations Fighting AIDS) provided insightful context into the use of death-sentence messaging in posters, as well as how the move away from such messaging was enabled by activists who promoted public health practices on their own terms. Advocates' response to government messaging can be seen in the posters created by AIDeS (explored by Jessica Lacher-Feldman), as well as "Semen Kit" (Siân Cook) and "Stop the Church" (Tamar W. Carroll). The creators of the latter actively mobilized against the Catholic Church's rejection of sensible prevention methods in favor of doctrine.

Writers also chose posters from the revival of the medium beginning around 2010 when AIDS Action NOW! sponsored the PosterVirus project. This collective created and distributed new messages that echoed the political voice of the AIDS movement at a time when the broader public considered the crisis over. Stigma and criminalization as well as popular narratives of the AIDS "past" all came under attack as these posters appeared on urban streets. But absent the political movement of an earlier generation of activists, their impact remained discursive, their calls unanswered. Through our efforts on publishing this book, we hope to connect current posters to that past and to look to the present moment in which the HIV/AIDS crisis is far from over.

Ian Bradley-Perrin is a Ph.D. candidate in Sociomedical Sciences at Columbia University Mailman School of Public Health in New York City.

"AP" numbers and how to search the collection online

The entire collection of AIDS posters is available online at: https://aep.lib.rochester.edu/

Users are able to search and browse for poster information at this site. Each poster has a unique identifier, called an AP number, allowing each poster to be sorted, described, stored, and retrieved physically and online. If you know what poster you are looking for, by AP number, you can simply enter that AP number into search bar on the website. At the top of the site, there is also a "Browse" function which allows users to sort by country or by language, as well as some advanced search options. As the collection continues to grow, new posters will be added to the site, and additional metadata updated when appropriate. Assistance is available by contacting the University of Rochester's River Campus Libraries Department of Rare Books, Special Collections, and Preservation.

RAISING AWARENESS

"AIDS—Hidden Danger"

The artist group General Idea covered bus shelters, fences, and gallery walls with wallpaper, endlessly replicating this image to represent how AIDS spread and invaded private and public spaces. For me, "Imagevirus" remains an iconic expression of the virus itself and our efforts to reckon with it.

AA Bronson, Felix Partz, and Jorge Zontal, three artists who formed General Idea in Toronto in 1969, in the wake of the summer of love, and produced work that mirrored, disrupted, and challenged pop culture. This 1987 work marked a shift to addressing the impact of HIV, a subject they continued to explore until Partz's and Zontal's deaths from complications related to AIDS in 1994.

Like so many other artists addressing AIDS, General Idea took something familiar and changed its perspective. Robert Indiana's cheery, ubiquitous, hippie-era "LOVE" became "AIDS" (forcing one to consider that connection), multiplying and transforming everything it touches. Its familiarity might be unnoticed by those who sped by it and unavoidable for those who were forced to confront it regularly. Eventually we all had to acknowledge it.

"Imagevirus," the wallpaper that multiplied this design, is one of the ways that AIDS activists and artists (a narrow distinction) were able to insert AIDS into the public sphere and the public conversation. Borrowing and subverting the language of advertising and pop culture, activists used the master's tools to demand that the house be rebuilt and that one of its many rooms be adapted for our needs. In other words, AIDS took something all too familiar, and by shifting orientation, changed our perspective.

Karen Herland

Karen Herland is an activist, organizer, and educator currently teaching at Concordia University's Interdisciplinary Major in Sexuality Studies in Montréal.

"AIDS," 1987
New York, New York, U.S.A.
Creators: Koury Wingate
Designer: General Idea
(after Robert Indiana's "LOVE" design)
80 x 80 cm
AP1938

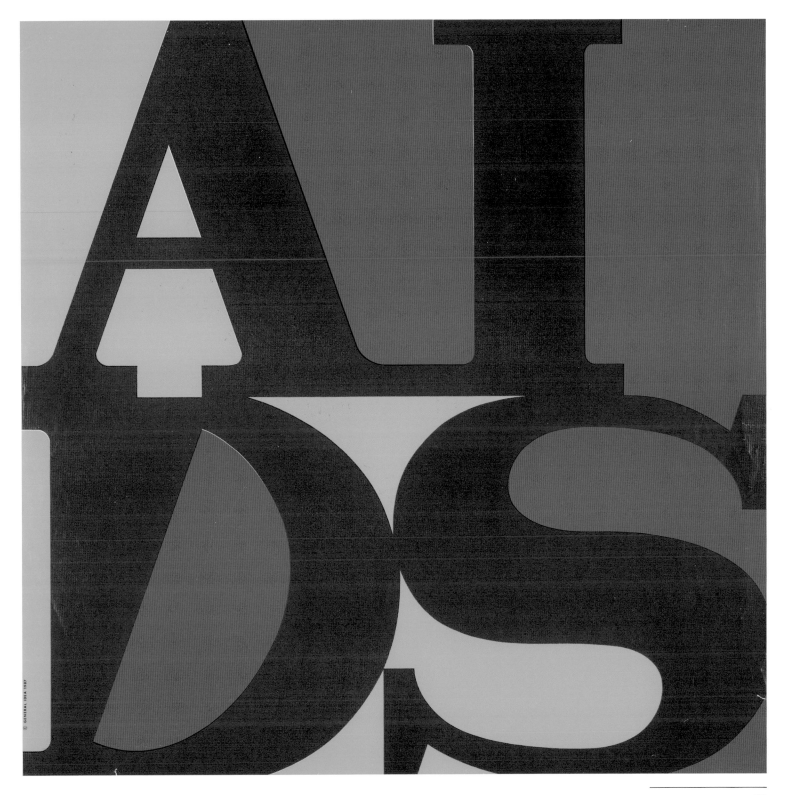

© GENERAL IDEA 1987

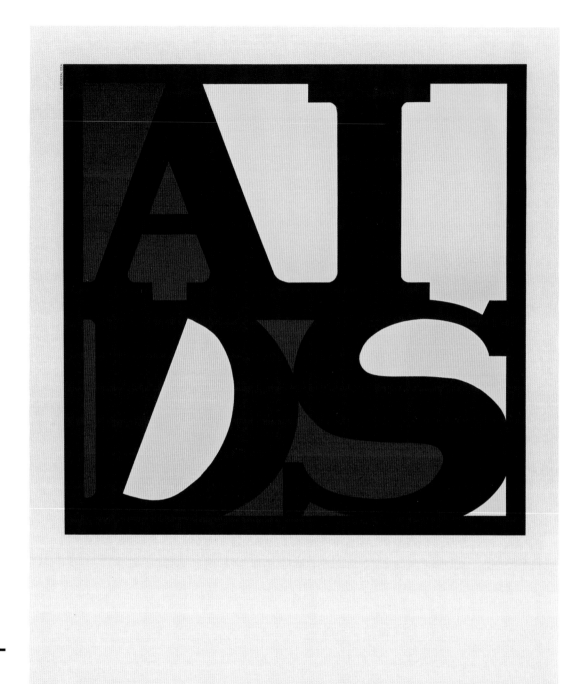

Arbeitsgemeinschaft deutscher AIDS-STIFTUNGEN

"AIDS," n.d.
Germany
Creator: Arbeitsgemeinschaft Deutscher
AIDS-Stiftungen
Designer: General Idea
(after Robert Indiana's "LOVE" design)
60 x 42 cm
AP5980

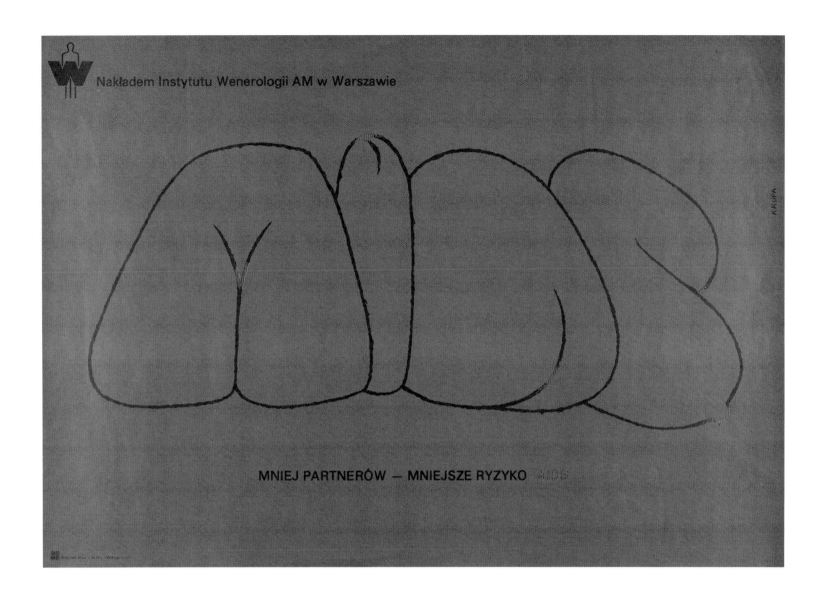

"AIDS. Fewer Partners—Less Risk"
(translated from Polish), n.d.
Poland
Creator: Instytutu Wenerologi
AM w Warszawie
47 x 66 cm
AP50013

"AIDS—Hidden Danger," 2006
U.S.A.
Designer: Čedomir Kostović
68 x 99 cm
AP50039

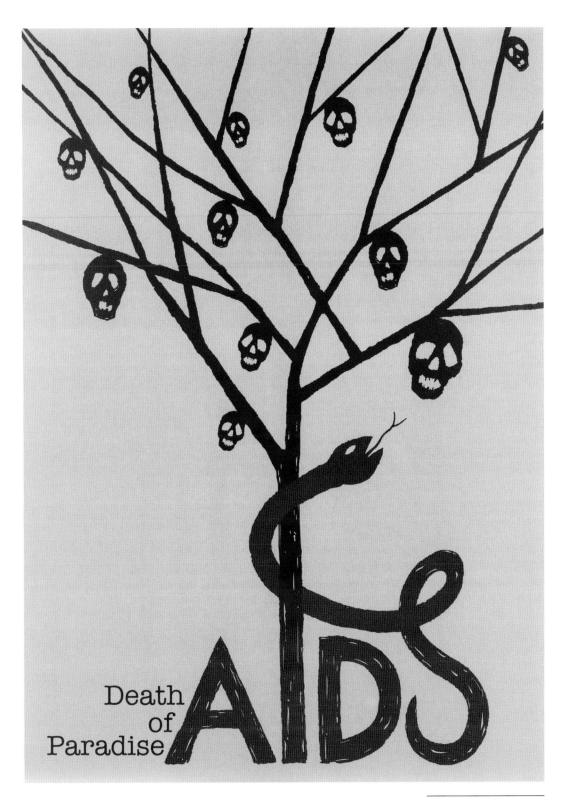

"AIDS: Death of Paradise," ca. 2000
South Korea
Designer: Sang-Rak Kim
104 x 73 cm
AP50028

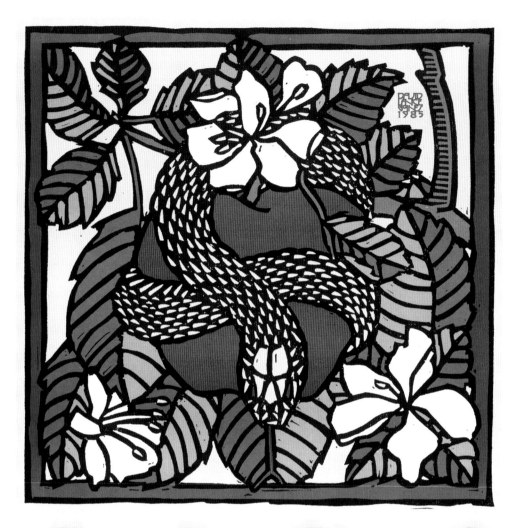

"AIDS Prevention," 1985
Berkeley, California, U.S.A.
Creator: University of California, Berkeley,
Student Health Service
Designer: David Lance Goines
61 x 44 cm
AP205

The image is stark and static, but the experience of this campaign, bearing the tagline "AIDS does not forgive," was a turning point in the experience of COCQ-SIDA (Coalition des organismes communautaires québécois de lutte contre le SIDA), on the social marketing front.

To be fair, this was never intended to be a poster. The campaign began as two television spots, one straight and one gay, each beginning with a tight focus on bodies writhing in pleasure. As the camera pulls back, it reveals that the "action" is taking place in a coffin. Both couples are very much alive and still writhing at the end of their respective spots. Still, they were focused on the "death" message, which was in direct contradiction with the work that COCQ-SIDA and its member groups were doing (and continue to do) to support the inclusion of people living with HIV in the lives of their communities. Freezing the images into static posters reinforced the "death" message and further stymied the fight for inclusion.

It was much worse in context, as two other players in Québec society launched their own "death" message campaigns the same year.

The Ministry of Health and Social Services issued a series of posters depicting graveyard monuments focusing on the three target populations (gay men, heterosexuals, and people who inject drugs) with the tagline "Le SIDA circule toujours" ("AIDS Always Gets Around"). The Comité des personnes atteintes du VIH du Québec (CPAVIH, since closed) had a poster campaign showing the headboards of beds in a cemetery.

The death message couldn't have been clearer, or more rejected by, the community of people living with HIV. From then on, the COCQ-SIDA Board of Directors resolved not to accept campaigns proposed by ad agencies without having had a hand in their messaging. First, we tried reactively to tweak the imagery and the messages, and ever since, we have proactively written a brief outlining our expectations.

Ken Monteith

Ken Monteith is executive director of COCQ-SIDA, the Québec coalition of AIDS organizations, based in Montréal.

Untitled, ca. 2004
Montreal, Québec, Canada
Creator: Coalition des organismes communautaires québécois de lutte contre le SIDA
91 x 61 cm
AP2481

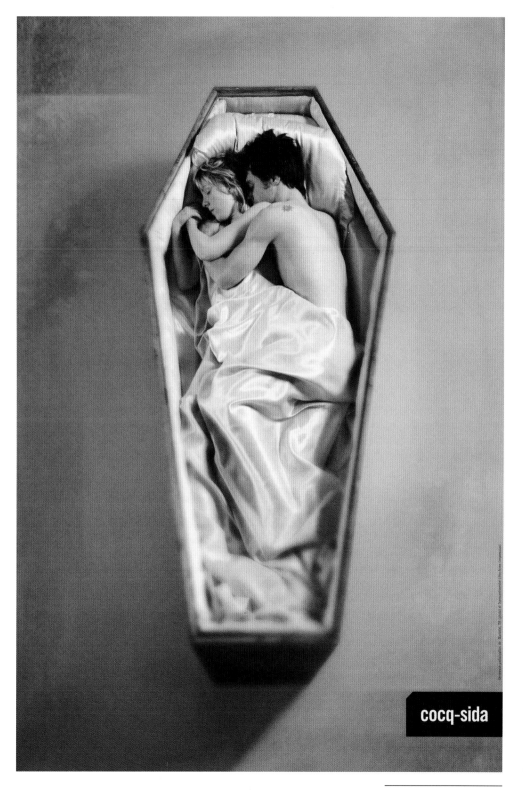

"Get the Answers. Ask about AIDS," n.d.
Boston, Massachusetts, U.S.A.
Creator: AIDS Action Committee of
Massachusetts
Designer: Katherine Shorey
71 x 51 cm
AP1906

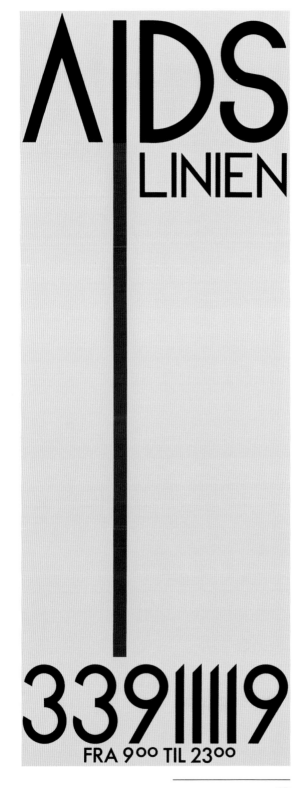

"AIDS-Line" (translated from Danish), n.d.
Copenhagen, Denmark
Creator: AIDS-Linien
59 x 22 cm
AP3886

Si eres VIH positivo o tienes el SIDA,
¡Llámanos!

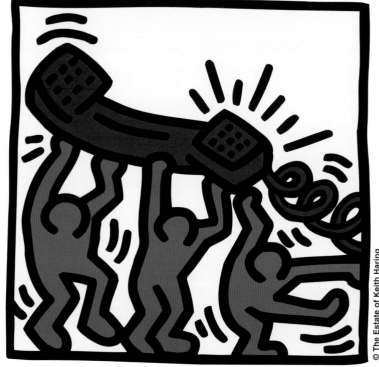

1-800-TALK-HIV
1 - 8 0 0 - 8 2 5 - 5 4 4 8
La Línea Informativa sobre el SIDA
El Departamento de Salud de la Ciudad de Nueva York

| Rudolph W. Giuliani | Benjamin Mojica, M.D., M.P.H |
| Alcalde | Comisionado Interino |

Printing made possible by a grant from the "Ryan White CARE Act Title I" U.S. Health Resources and Services Administration

"If You Are HIV Positive or Have AIDS,
Call Us!" (translated from Spanish), n.d.
New York, New York, U.S.A.
Creator: New York City
Department of Health
Designer: Keith Haring
56 x 54 cm
AP1173

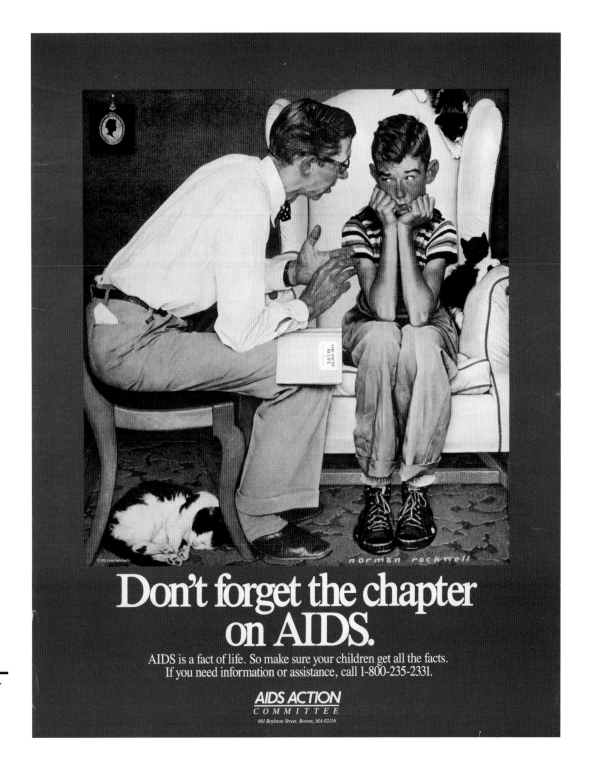

"Don't Forget the Chapter on AIDS," 1987
Boston, Massachusetts, U.S.A.
Creator: AIDS Action Committee
of Massachusetts
Illustration: Norman Rockwell
64 x 49 cm
AP799

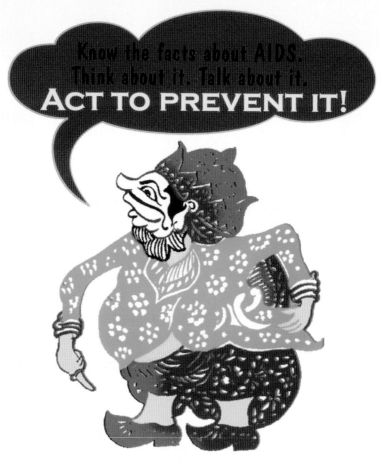

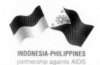

"Know the Facts about AIDS. Think about It.
Talk about It. Act to Prevent It!" 2001
Indonesia
Creator: Indonesia-Philippines
Partnership against AIDS
33 x 25 cm
AP3661

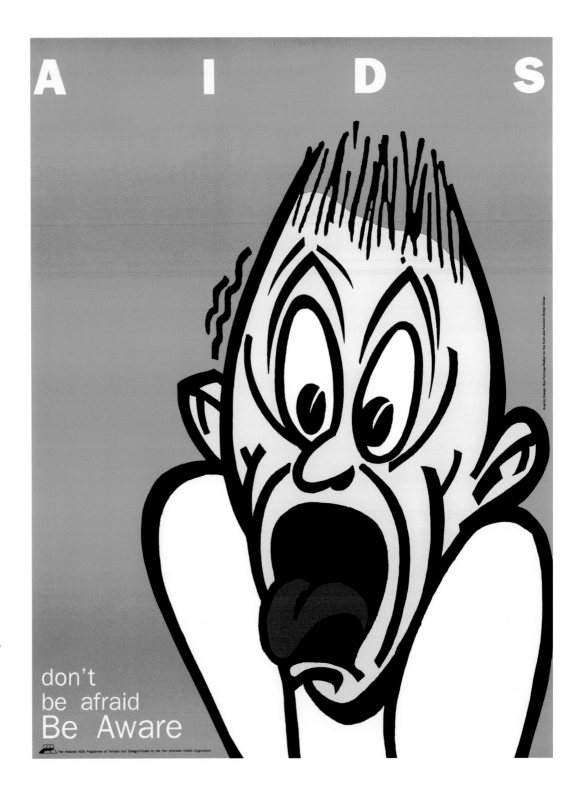

"AIDS. Don't Be Afraid. Be Aware,"
ca. 1994
Trinidad and Tobago
Creator: National AIDS Programme
of Trinidad and Tobago
Designer: Illya Furlonge-Walker for the
Form and Function Design Group
60 x 42 cm
AP3004

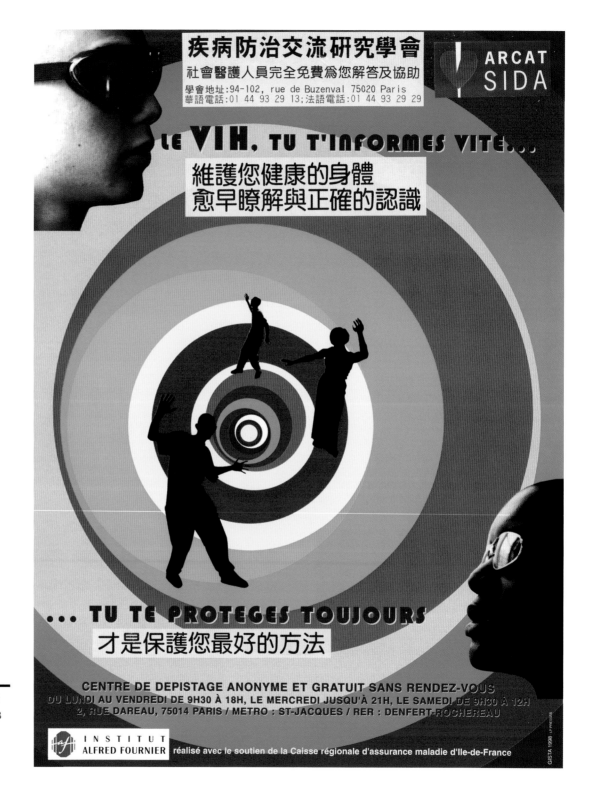

"HIV. Get Informed Fast...Always Protect
Yourself" (translated from French), 1998
Paris, France
Creator: ARCAT
77 x 56 cm
AP6534

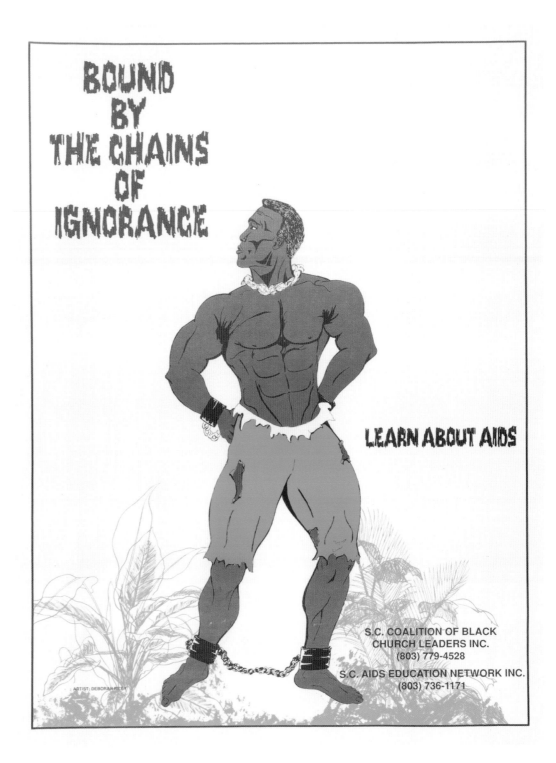

"Bound by the Chains of Ignorance.
Learn about AIDS," n.d.
South Carolina, U.S.A.
Creator: South Carolina Coalition of Black
Church Leaders, South Carolina AIDS
Education Network
61 x 46 cm
AP1630

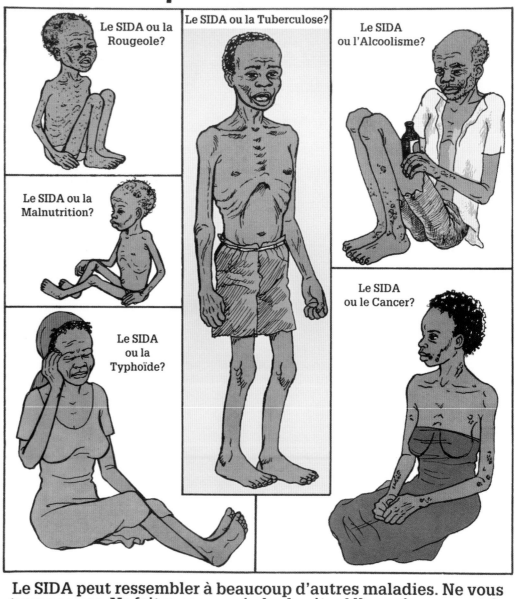

A quoi ressemble une personne qui a le SIDA?

Le SIDA ou la Rougeole?

Le SIDA ou la Tuberculose?

Le SIDA ou l'Alcoolisme?

Le SIDA ou la Malnutrition?

Le SIDA ou la Typhoïde?

Le SIDA ou le Cancer?

Le SIDA peut ressembler à beaucoup d'autres maladies. Ne vous trompez pas. Ne faites pas courir des bruits. Allez voir un agent de santé qualifié pour faire des tests si vous pensez que vous avez le SIDA ou que quelqu'un que vous connaissez a peut-être le SIDA.

Ouganda Ecole de Santé. Matériel pour le Contrôle du SIDA (Item 5)
Ministère de l'Éducation, Ministère de la Santé (Programme de Contrôle du SIDA), UNICEF Kampala

"What Does a Person with AIDS Look Like?" (translated from French), ca. 1993
Series: *Uganda School Health Kit on AIDS Control*
Kampala, Uganda
Creator: Uganda Ministry of Health, AIDS Control Programme
60 x 42 cm
AP3417

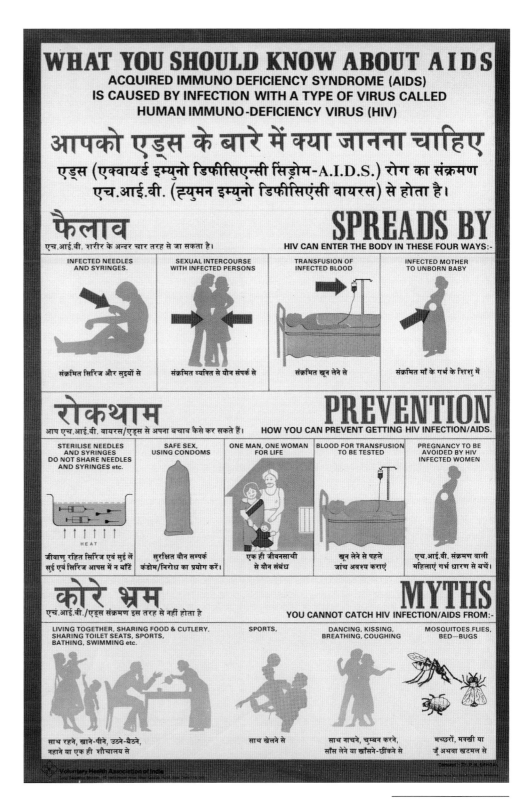

"What You Should Know about AIDS," n.d.
New Delhi, India
Creator: Voluntary Health Association
of India
73 x 49 cm
AP3674

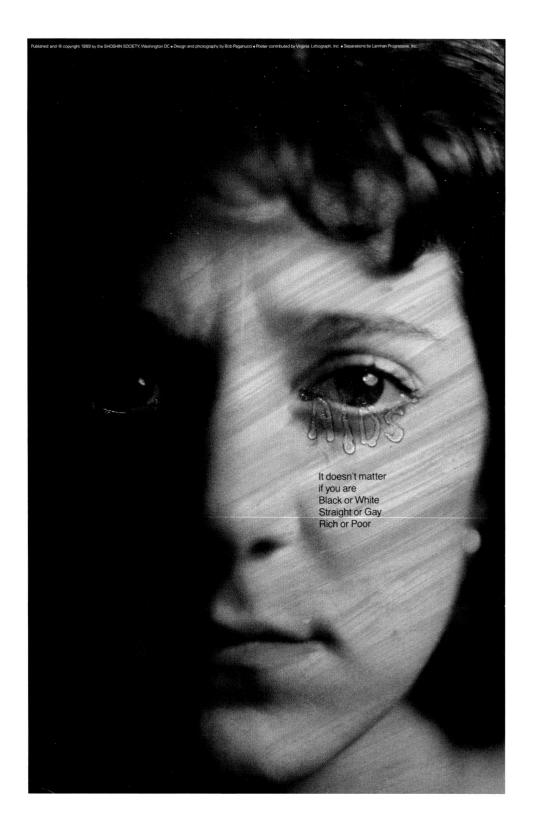

It doesn't matter
if you are
Black or White
Straight or Gay
Rich or Poor

"AIDS. It Doesn't Matter If You Are Black
or White, Straight or Gay, Rich or Poor,"
1989
District of Columbia, U.S.A.
Creator: Shoshin Society
Designer: Robert Paganucci
62 x 40 cm
AP554

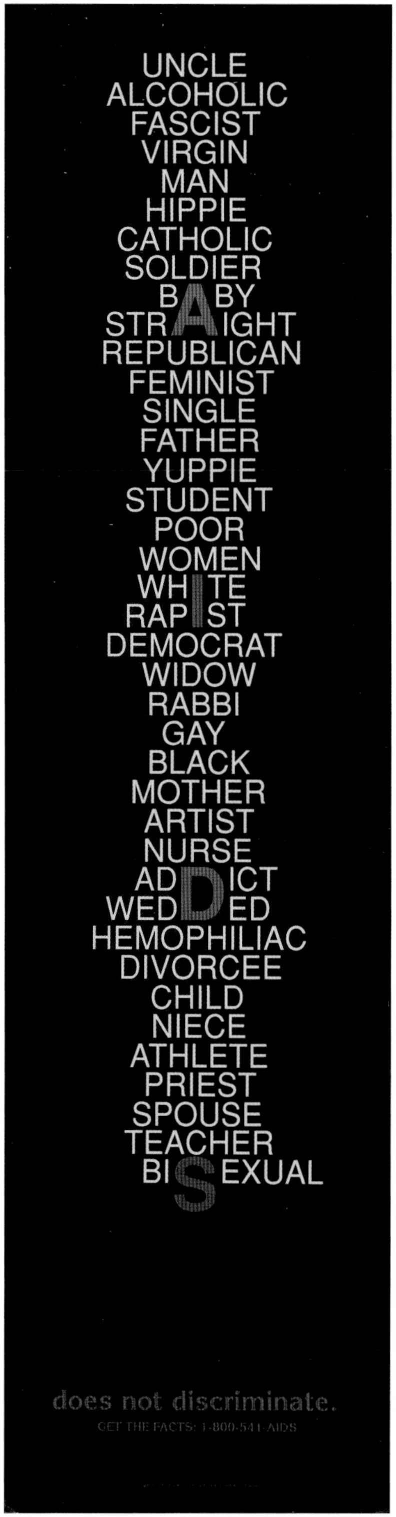

UNCLE
ALCOHOLIC
FASCIST
VIRGIN
MAN
HIPPIE
CATHOLIC
SOLDIER
B**A**BY
STR**A**IGHT
REPUBLICAN
FEMINIST
SINGLE
FATHER
YUPPIE
STUDENT
POOR
WOMEN
WH**I**TE
RAP**I**ST
DEMOCRAT
WIDOW
RABBI
GAY
BLACK
MOTHER
ARTIST
NURSE
AD**D**ICT
WED**D**ED
HEMOPHILIAC
DIVORCEE
CHILD
NIECE
ATHLETE
PRIEST
SPOUSE
TEACHER
BI**S**EXUAL

does not discriminate.
GET THE FACTS: 1-800-541-AIDS

"AIDS Does Not Discriminate.
Get the Facts," n.d.
New York, New York, U.S.A.
Creator: New York State
Department of Health
95 x 25 cm
AP5230

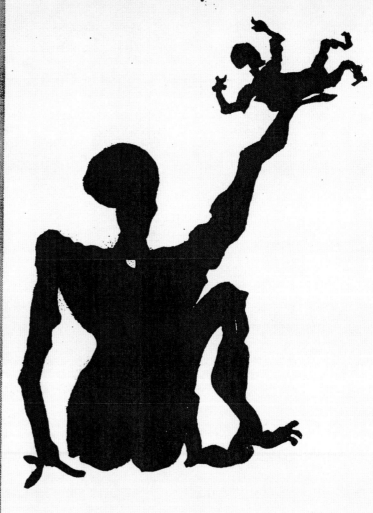

AIDS DOES NOT DISCRIMINATE

According to the Minority AIDS Project, California Department of Health Services:

51% of Women with AIDS are African-American.

25% of Women with AIDS are Latina.

57% of all children with AIDS are African-American.

25% of all AIDS cases are people of African-American descent.

14% of all AIDS cases are people of Latin-American descent.

OUR GOVERNMENT DISCRIMINATES AGAINST PEOPLE WITH AIDS

"AIDS Does Not Discriminate.
Our Government Discriminates against
People with AIDS," n.d.
California, U.S.A.
Creator: ACT UP
28 x 22 cm
AP387

YOU CAN GET AIDS

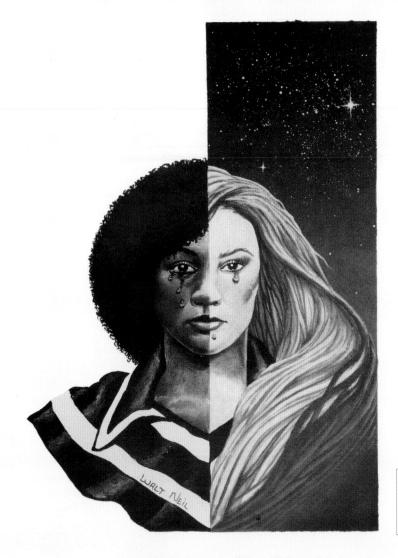

WALT NEIL

AIDS Does Not Discriminate

For Information About
AIDS Contact
The Urban League
or call 1-800-332-AIDS

0982.11

"You Can Get AIDS.
AIDS Does Not Discriminate," 1988
Ohio, U.S.A.
Creator: Ohio Department of Health
Designer: Walt Neil
36 x 28 cm
AP1398

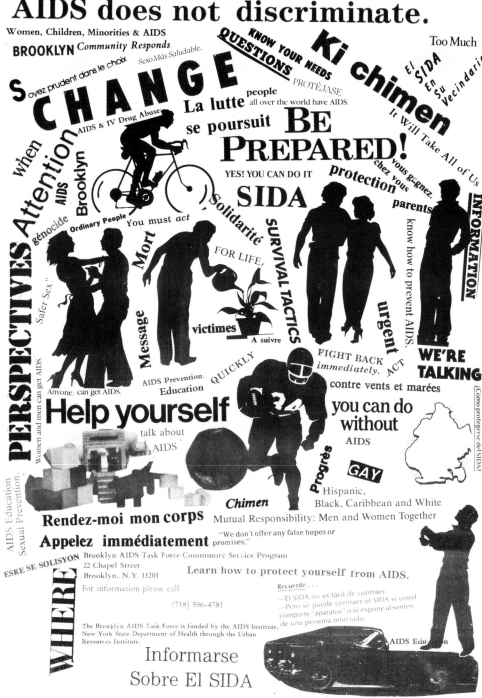

"AIDS Does Not Discriminate," n.d.
Brooklyn, New York, U.S.A.
Creator: Brooklyn AIDS Task Force
59 x 44 cm
AP1202

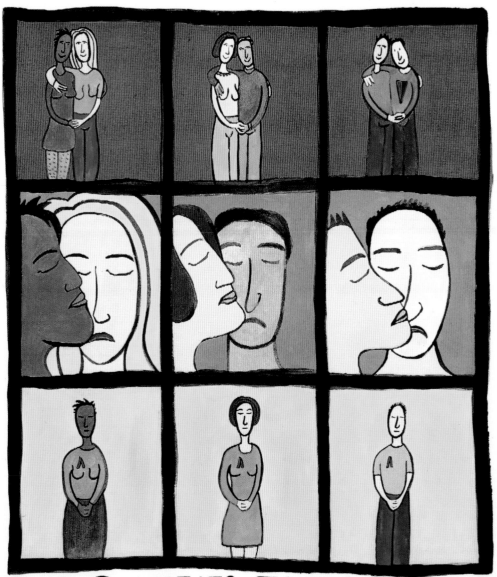

"AIDS Affects Everybody," 1995
Victoria, Australia
Creator: Victorian AIDS Council
Designer: Barbara Graham
60 x 42 cm
AP3180

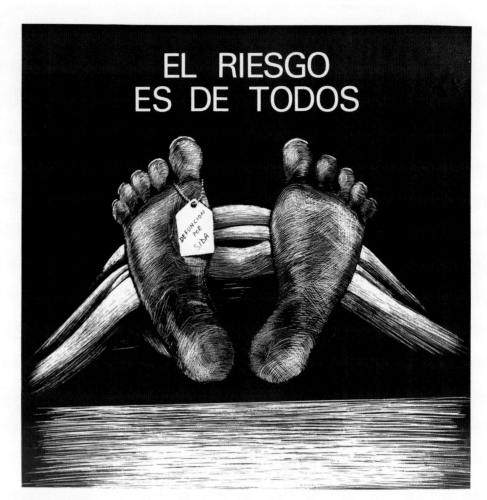

"Risk Belongs to Everyone.
If AIDS Happens"
(translated from Spanish), n.d.
Mexico City, Mexico
Creator: Consejo Nacional de Prevención
y Control del SIDA
61 x 40 cm
AP4382

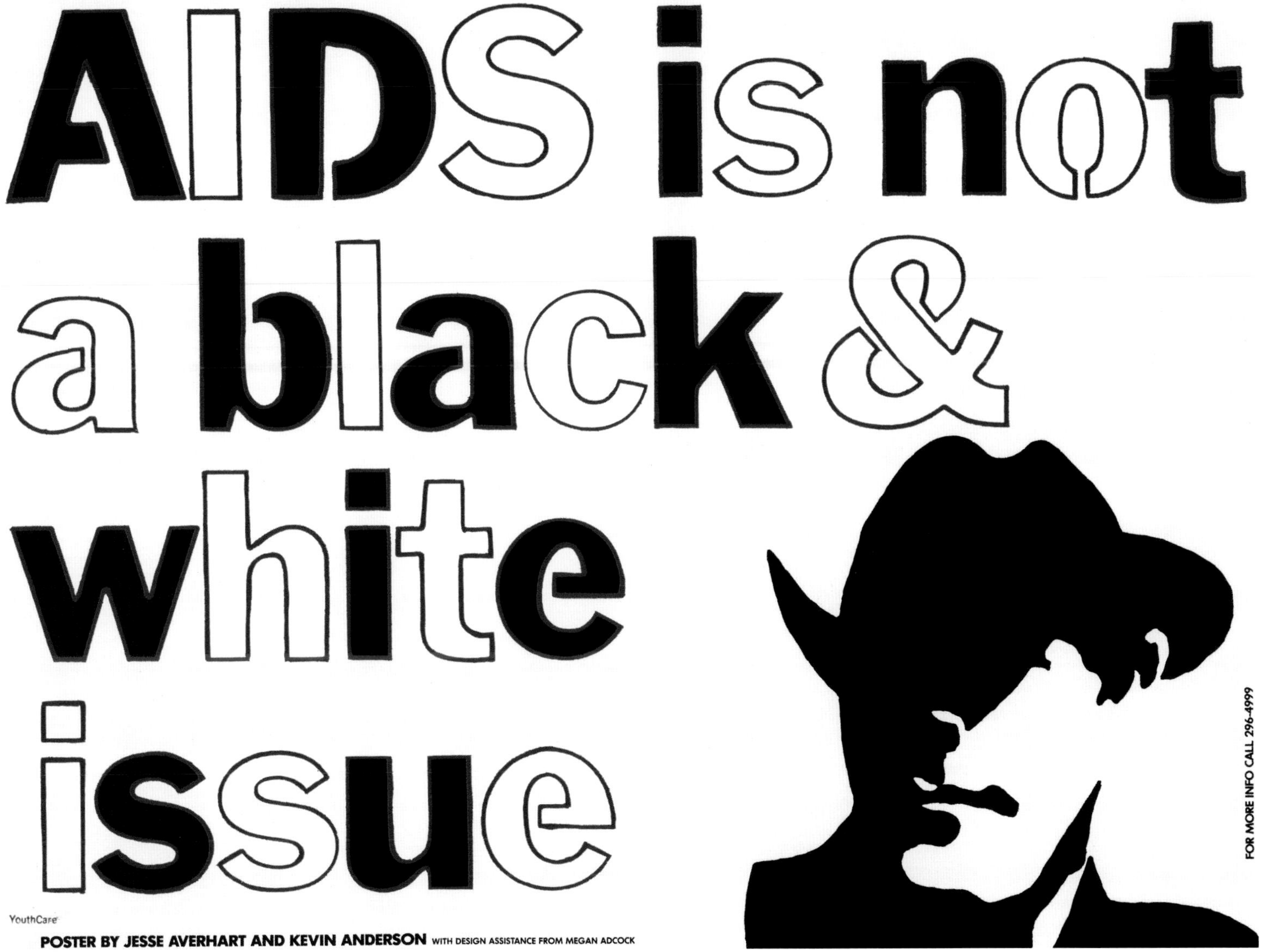

AIDS is not a black & white issue

YouthCare

POSTER BY JESSE AVERHART AND KEVIN ANDERSON WITH DESIGN ASSISTANCE FROM MEGAN ADCOCK

FOR MORE INFO CALL 296-4999

"AIDS Is Not a Black & White Issue," n.d.
Seattle, Washington, U.S.A.
Creator: YouthCare
Designers: Jesse Averhart and Kevin
Anderson with design assistance from
Megan Adcock
43 x 56 cm
AP1743

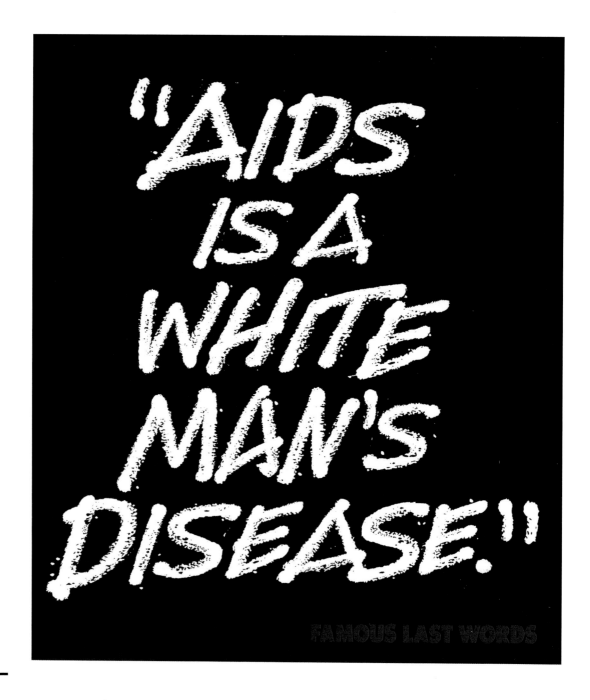

"AIDS Is a White Man's Disease. Famous Last Words," n.d.
Seattle, Washington, U.S.A.
Creator: People of Color against AIDS Network
43 x 30 cm
AP1668

Anyone can get AIDS. Find out how to prevent it. Call today.
PEOPLE OF COLOR AGAINST AIDS.
INFORMATION 296-4999.

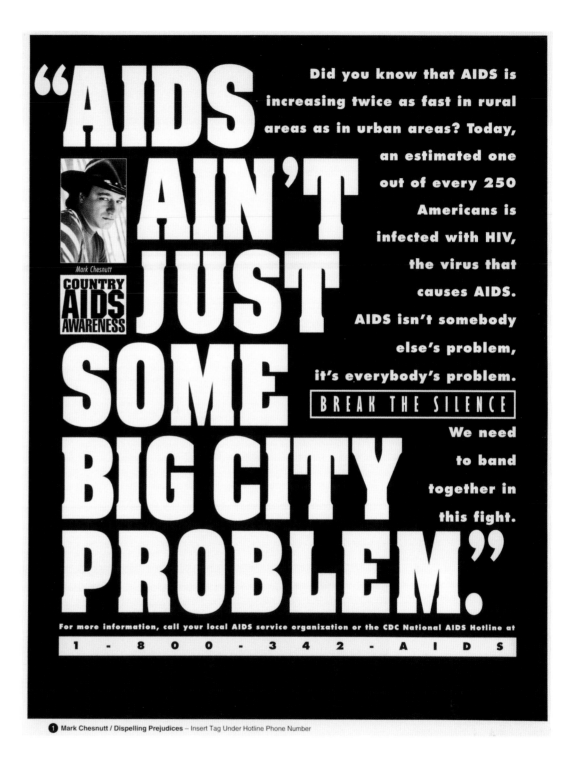

"AIDS Ain't Just Some Big City Problem,"
[singer-songwriter Mark Chesnutt], n.d.
Nashville, Tennessee, U.S.A.
Creator: Country AIDS
Awareness Campaign
30 x 23 cm
AP1595

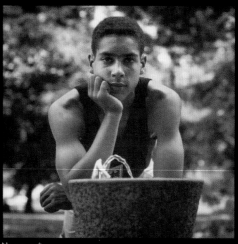

"Can You Get AIDS from a Drinking
  Fountain?" 1988
Toronto, Ontario, Canada
Creator: Ontario Ministry of Health
and Long-Term Care
63 x 41 cm
AP8028

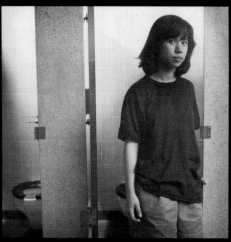

"Can You Get AIDS from a Toilet Seat?"
1988
Toronto, Ontario, Canada
Creator: Ontario Ministry of Health
and Long-Term Care
63 x 41 cm
AP4668

AIDS - What to know

Mosquito bites don't cause AIDS

You don't get AIDS in public places.

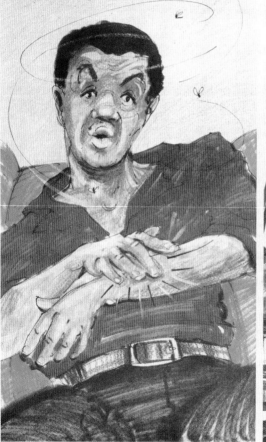

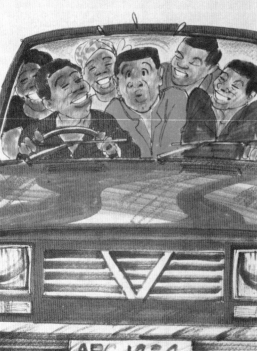

Ministry of Health, Nairobi, Kenya.

"AIDS—What to Know," n.d.
Nairobi, Kenya
Creator: National AIDS and STDs
Control Programme
60 x 42 cm
AP3457

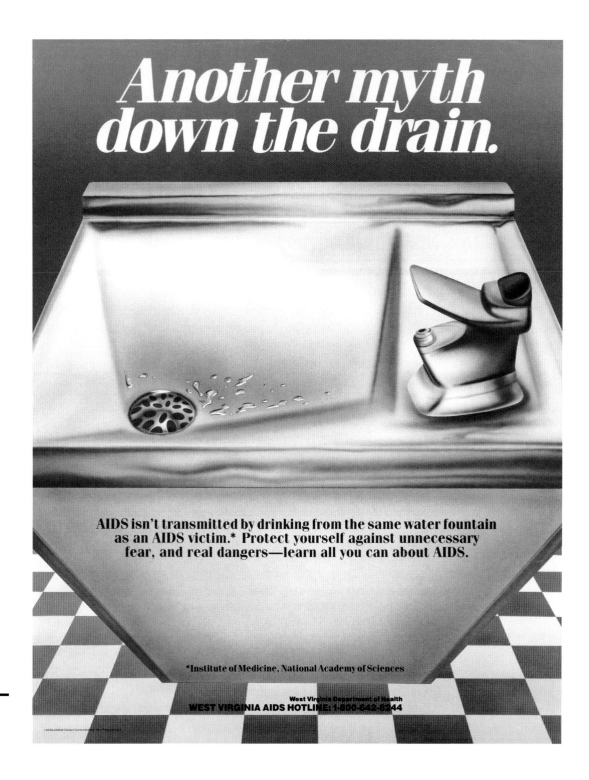

"Another Myth Down the Drain," 1988
Charleston, West Virginia, U.S.A.
Creator: West Virginia State
Department of Health
56 x 43 cm
AP1749

KISSING DOESN'T KILL: GREED AND INDIFFERENCE DO.

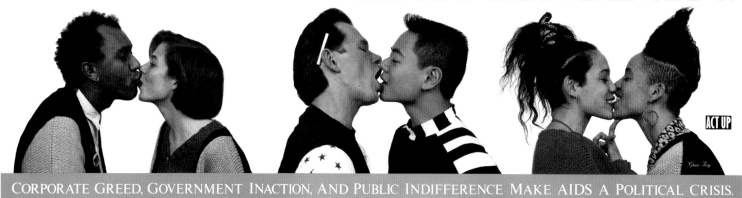

CORPORATE GREED, GOVERNMENT INACTION, AND PUBLIC INDIFFERENCE MAKE AIDS A POLITICAL CRISIS.

"Kissing Doesn't Kill:
Greed and Indifference Do," 1989–90
New York, New York, U.S.A.
Creator: amfAR as part of
"Art on the Road"
Designer: Gran Fury
29 x 94 cm
AP5165

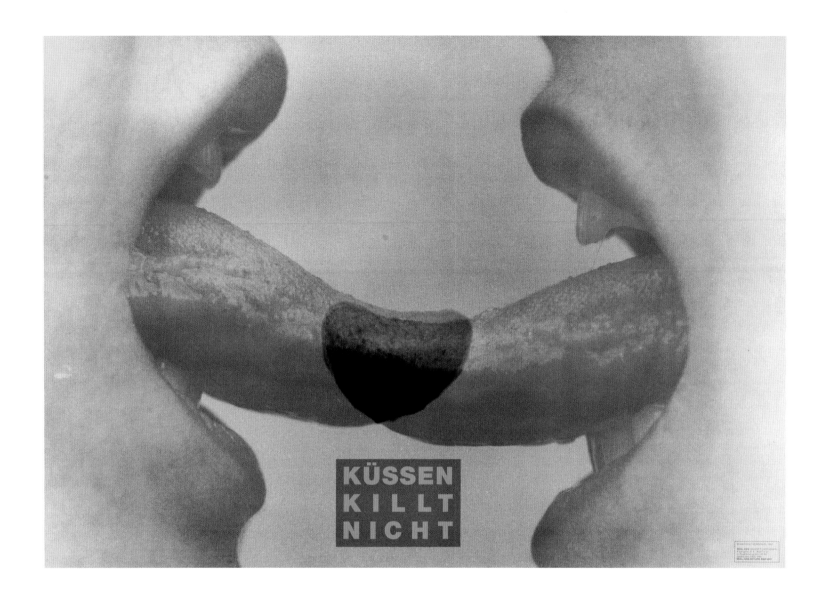

"Kissing Doesn't Kill"
(translated from German), 1993
Graz, Austria
Creator: Real AIDS Grazer Kunstverein
in cooperation with the Steirischen
AIDS-Hilfe
Designer: Mathias Herrmann
60 x 84 cm
AP5894

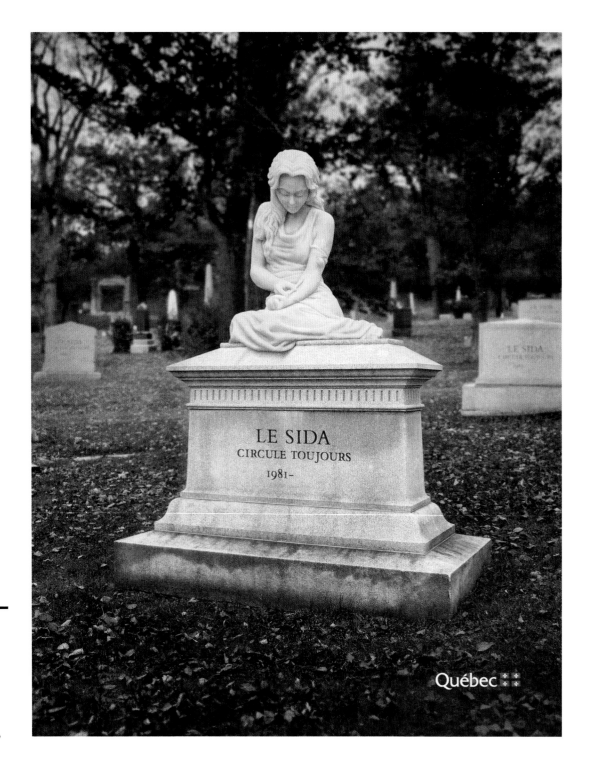

"AIDS Always Gets Around: 1981–"
(translated from French), 2004
Montreal, Québec, Canada
Creator: Province of Québec,
Ministère de la santé et des
services sociaux. Centre québécois
de coordination sur le SIDA
Designer: MARKETEL, Gilles Dusablon,
Linda Dawe, Stephane Gaulin
43 x 33 cm
AP5312

AIDS is over, right?

(or maybe, you should read the fine print)

One in four people who become infected with HIV is under the age of 20. In 1997, 55% of Americans wrongly believed they could become infected by sharing a glass of water, up from 48% in '91. Ignorance is bliss. 29% of Americans living with HIV have no health insurance. ADAP (AIDS Drug Assistance Program) is bankrupt in over half of the 50 states, which means that they cannot provide access to the protease cocktail. The protease cocktail costs $16,000 per year per person. Ignorance is bliss. Unprotected sex is the main risk behavior amongst teenagers, accounting for 55% of reported HIV infections in young men, and 37% in young women, as of 1996. While 95% of Americans believe that public schools should provide HIV prevention education, frank discussion of sexuality and condoms in the classroom is still virtually taboo. Ignorance is bliss. Last year, 41% of Americans wrongly believed they could contract HIV from a public toilet, up from 34% in '91 Ignorance is bliss. AIDS deaths are down. Transmission is up. More people are living with AIDS. Nearly half of HIV+ people undergoing triple-combination therapy have developed resistance, rendering the drugs useless. Ignorance is bliss. One person is infected with HIV in the US every 13 minutes. Ignorance is bliss. 33 Americans are infected every day due to lack of access to needle-exchange programs. 66% of Americans approve of needle-exchange programs, yet the government has maintained the ban on funding for needle-exchange. Ignorance is bliss. More than 40% of AIDS cases worldwide are among women. 16,000 people become infected with HIV every day. By the year 2000, there will be more than 40 million people living with HIV/AIDS worldwide. AIDS is over, right?

DAY WITHOUT ART December 1, 1998

the tenth international day of action and mourning in response to the AIDS crisis

A project of Visual AIDS: 526 west 26th street no. 510, ny, ny 10001 usa • phone 212.627.9855 • fax 212.627.9815 • e-mail: visAIDS@aol.com • Supporters of Visual AIDS in 1998: Con Edison, The Debs Foundation, The Geraldine R. Dodge Foundation, The Elton John AIDS Foundation, The Estate Project for Artists with AIDS, The Robert D. Farber Foundation, The Horace W. Goldsmith Foundation, The Mary J. Hutchins Foundation, Materials for the Arts, The National Endowment for the Arts, individual donors and all DAY WITHOUT ART participants. With thanks to APICHA, The Door, Lower East Side Harm Reduction Center, People With AIDS Health Group, School's Out: The Naming Project, and SLAAAP!. Digital Pre-Press/Production: Katz Digital Technologies Inc. (NY)   Printing: Louis Sherman & Co.

"AIDS Is Over, Right?" 1998
Series: *Day without Art*
New York, New York, U.S.A.
Creator: Visual AIDS
89 x 60 cm
AP5229

"AIDS Is a Women's Issue"

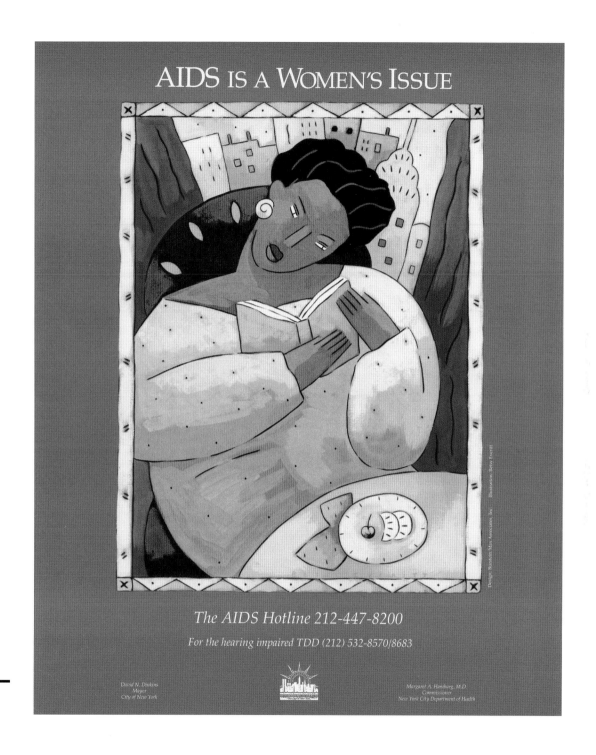

"AIDS Is a Women's Issue," 1990–1993
New York, New York, U.S.A.
Creator: New York City
Department of Health
Designer: Betsy Everitt
71 x 28 cm
AP1072

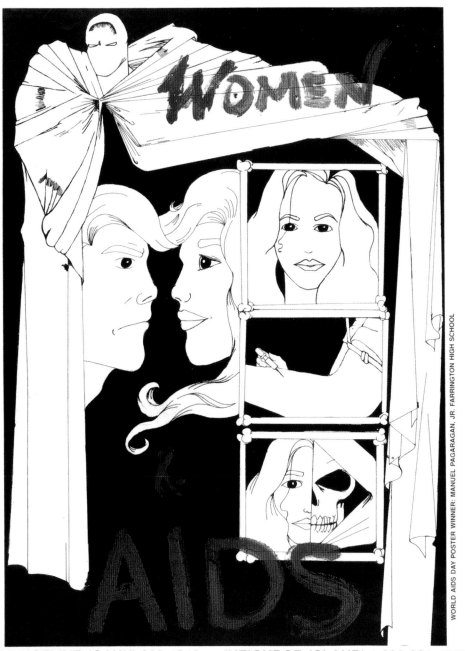

WORLD AIDS DAY POSTER WINNER: MANUEL PAGARAGAN, JR. FARRINGTON HIGH SCHOOL

AIDS HOTLINE (OAHU) 922-1313   (NEIGHBOR ISLAND) 1-800-321-1555

"Women & AIDS," n.d.
Oahu, Hawaii, U.S.A.
Creator: AIDS Hotline
Designer: Manuel Pagaragan, Jr.,
Farrington High School
51 x 41 cm
AP623

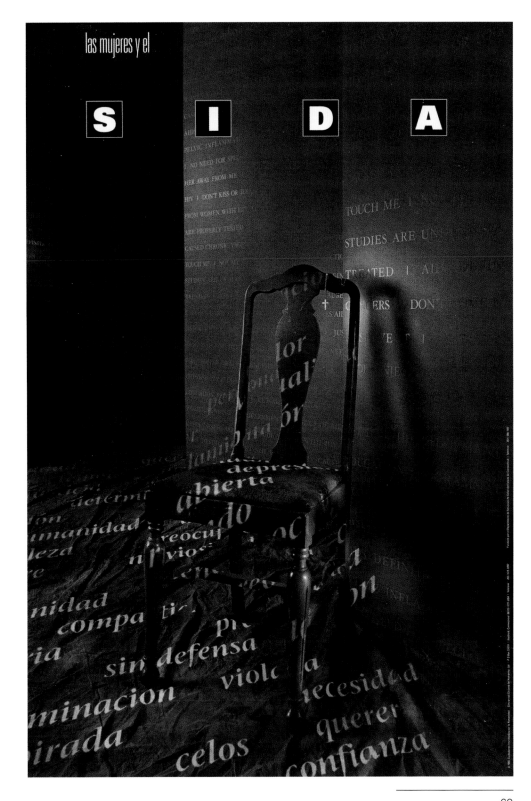

"Women and AIDS"
(translated from Spanish), 1992
Hartford, Connecticut, U.S.A.
Creator: Concerned Citizens
for Humanity
69 x 46 cm
AP496

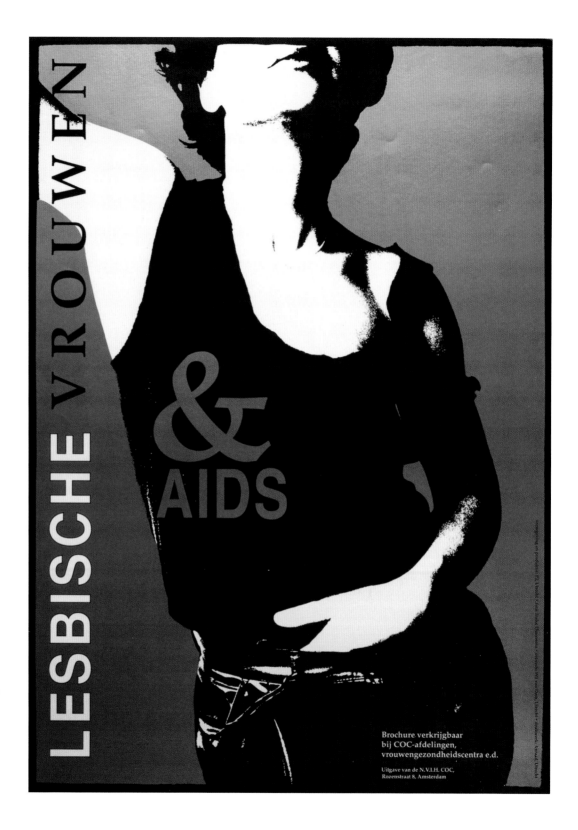

"Lesbians & AIDS"
(translated from Dutch), 1991
Amsterdam, Netherlands
Creator: COC Nederland
60 x 42 cm
AP5636

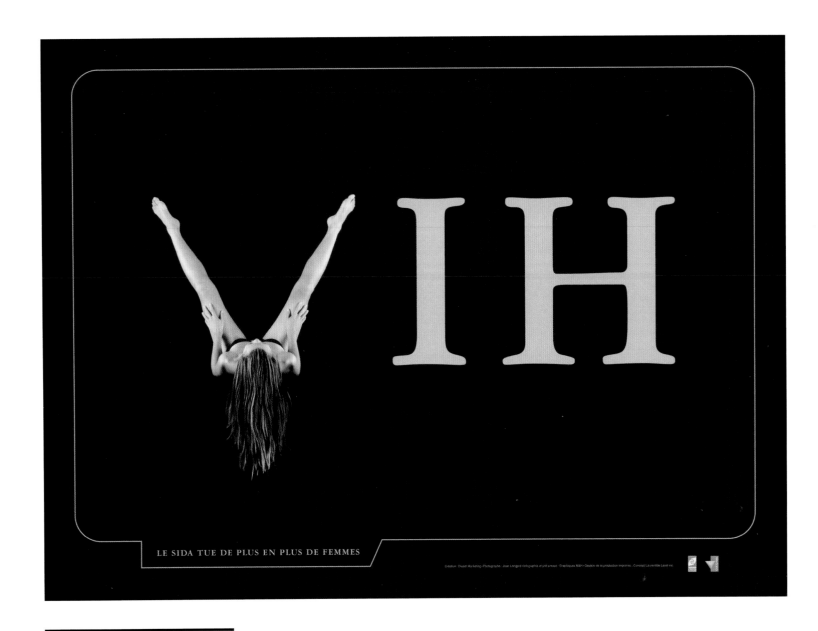

"HIV: AIDS Is Killing More and More
Women" (translated from French), 2001
Montreal, Québec, Canada
Creator: Comité des personnes
atteintes du VIH du Québec
Designer: Diesel Marketing with info-
graphics by M&H and photograph by
Jean Longpré
46 x 61 cm
AP2553

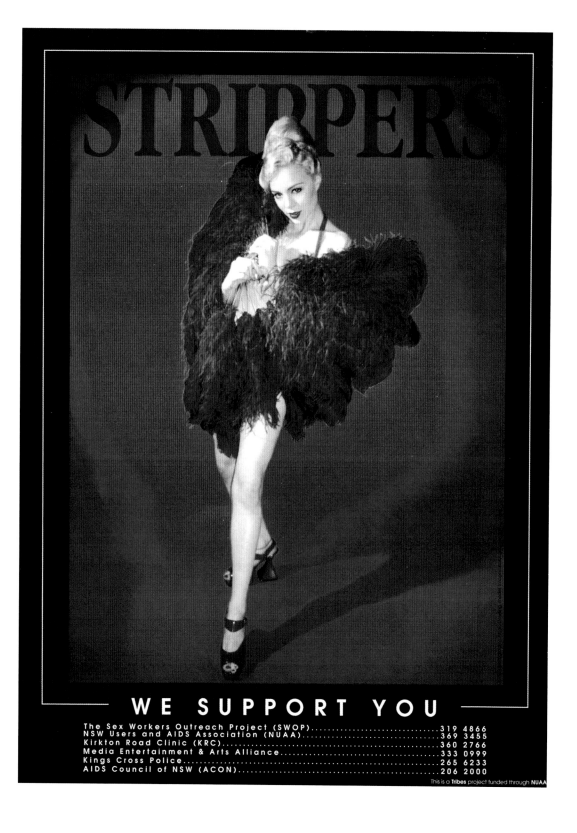

"Strippers: We Support You," n.d.
New South Wales, Australia
Creator: New South Wales
Users and AIDS Association
58 x 42 cm
AP3312

"AIDS. A Worldwide Effort Will Stop It"

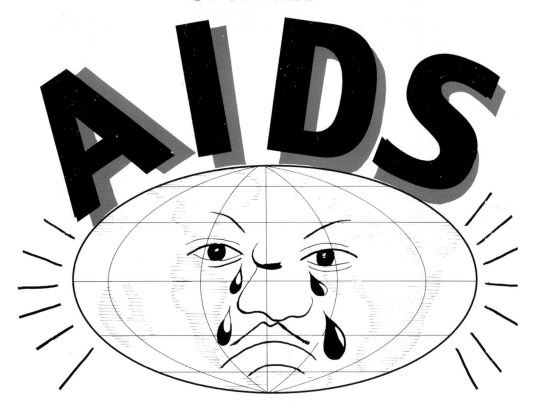

THE WORLD GROANS UNDER

AIDS

CURB THE SPREAD OF AIDS

worldview - kenya
Nairobi

THE FORD FOUNDATION
Office of East Africa

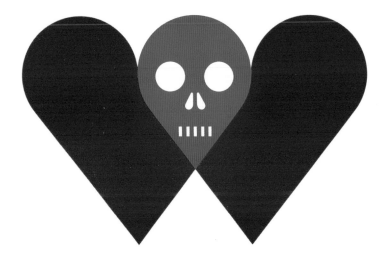

AIDS
A worldwide effort will stop it.

WORLD HEALTH ORGANIZATION
SPECIAL PROGRAMME ON AIDS

"AIDS. A Worldwide Effort Will Stop It,"
1987
Creator: WHO, Special Programme
on AIDS
Designer: Milton Glaser
92 x 61 cm
AP6781

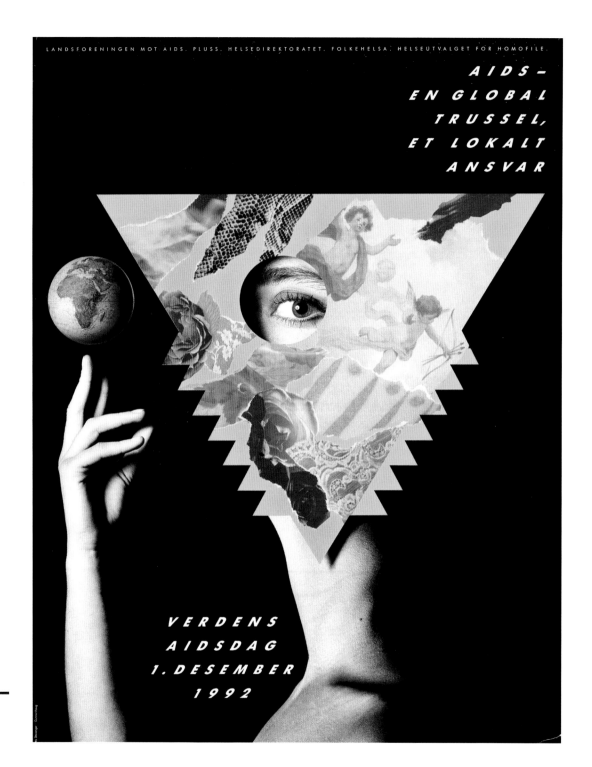

"AIDS: A Global Threat, A Local Answer"
(translated from Norwegian), 1992
Norway
Creator: Landsforeningen Mot AIDS
65 x 50 cm
AP3909

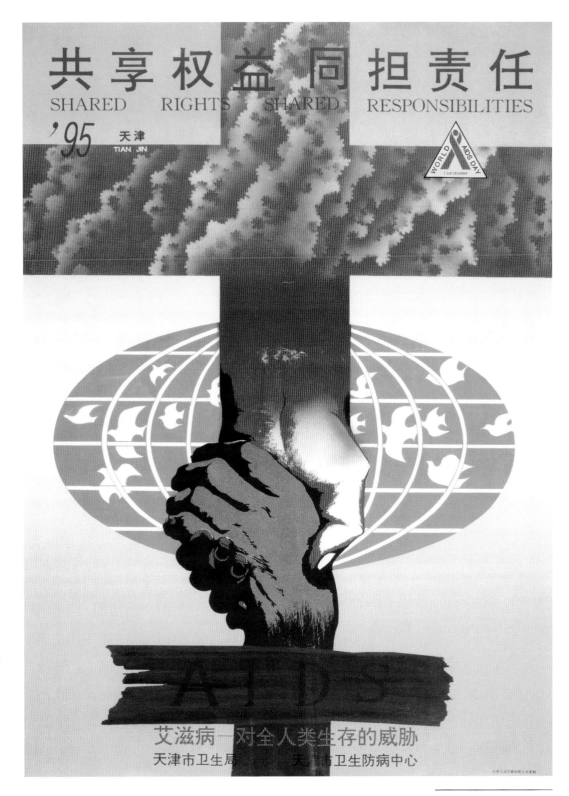

"Shared Rights. Shared Responsibilities,"
1995
China
Creator: Chinese Association of STD and
AIDS Control and Prevention
53 x 38 cm
AP3822

This is a poster from a candlelight vigil for World AIDS Day in 1989. The poster is stylized, and we can see only the flames. The poster is one of the last where one can see a whole community involved: government bodies, hospital wards dedicated to PLWHA, queer and other NGOs, memorial funds, and religious groups united to commemorate the ones lost or living with the virus. Later on, the community would fracture into different parts, a wound that still has not fully healed. Some of this era has been described in a trilogy written, and later televised, by the queer Swedish author Jonas Gardell, titled *Don't Ever Wipe Tears without Gloves*. In my research, I have interviewed men in San Francisco who described their raw and perpetual losses, how communities and contexts were shattered, and how they were left with ghosts. Twenty-five years later the losses were still there.

The poster is from a time when I myself was a budding "gayling," knowing that I wanted men but uncertain that I would survive. How long would it be until I was the dying one? More than two decades after having published my first article on gay men's health, I have seen the tremendous changes that have happened in queer rights in Sweden, even though issues remain. In my profession as a nurse, I was fortunate enough to meet not only the survivors in the initial NNRTI trial, but also the nurses and physicians who have cared at the front lines. HIV is now a treatable virus, and in some instances quite "unsexy" in Sweden, being the first country to reach the WHO's 90-90-90 target,[1] yet the stigma still remains and reappears when PLWHA (People Living with HIV/AIDS) need care in a facility.

Mats Christiansen

Mats Christiansen is a lecturer in nursing at Uppsala University, Sweden, and a Ph.D. candidate at Åbo Akademi University, Finland.

1. By 2020, 90% of all people living with HIV will know their HIV status, 90% of all people with diagnosed HIV infection will receive sustained antiretroviral therapy, and 90% of all people receiving antiretroviral therapy will have viral suppression. UNAIDS, "90-90-90 Treatment," https://www.unaids.org/en/resources/909090 (accessed March 23, 2020).

"Candle March" (translated from Swedish), 1989
Stockholm, Sweden
Creator: Noaks Ark-Roda korset
84 x 52 cm
AP4060

LJUS MARSCH

FREDAG 1 DECEMBER 1989

WORLD AIDS DAY

FÖR ATT MINNAS DE SOM AVLIDIT I AIDS OCH FÖR ATT VISA SOLIDARITET MED HIV-SMITTADE, AIDS-SJUKA, ANHÖRIGA OCH VÄNNER.
SAMLING KL 18.00 I KUNGSTRÄDGÅRDEN AVMARSCH KL 18.30 MINNESSTUND PÅ SERGELS TORG KL 19.00
MARSCHVÄG: KUNGSTRÄDGÅRDEN-VÄSTRA TRÄDGÅRDSGATAN-NORRLANDSGATAN-MÄSTER-SAMUELSGATAN-DROTTNINGGATAN-SERGELS TORG.

STIFTELSEN NOAKS ARK-RÖDA KORSET

I SAMARBETE MED AIDS-DELEGATIONEN · SVERIGES DÖVAS UNGDOMSRÅD · ESSEM-CENTER · FMN FÖRÄLDRAFÖRENINGEN MOT NARKOTIKA HEDVIG ELEONORA FÖRSAMLING · HOMOSEXUELLA JUDAR · HUDDINGE SJUKHUS FAMILJESOCIALA MOTTAGNINGEN PSYKIATRISKA KLINIK I KAROLINSKA SJUKHUSET HIV-MOTTAGNINGEN HUD-KLINIKEN · KISTA FÖRSAMLING · SVENSKA KOMMUNFÖRBUNDET · KUNGSHOLMS FÖRSAMLING · LANDSTINGET FÖREBYGGER AIDS · MARIA UNGDOMSENHET SAMTLIGA NOAKS ARK-FÖRENINGAR I SVERIGE · STIFTELSEN NORNA POSITIVA GRUPPEN STOCKHOLM · TIDNINGEN REPORTER · RFHL STOCKHOLM · RIKSFÖRBUNDET FÖR SEXUELLT LIKABERÄTTIGANDE RFSL · RFSU · ROSLAGSTULLS SJUKHUS · RÄDDA BARNENS RIKSFÖRBUND · SFS SVERIGES FÖRENADE STUDENTKÅRER · SOCIALSTYRELSEN - AIDS-KANSLIET · SKOLÖVERSTYRELSEN · STATENS BAKTERIOLOGISKA LABORATORIUM SBL · SÖDERSJUKHUSET AVDELNING 53 · SÖDERSJUKHUSET VENHÄLSAN · TEATERGRUPPEN EL GRILLO · SOCIALTJÄNSTEN STOCKHOLM · SVENSKA MISSIONSFÖRBUNDET · EKUMENISKA AIDSGRUPPEN · LÄKARE MOT AIDS · STIFTELSEN SIGHSTENS VÄNNER MOT AIDS · KAMRATFÖRENINGEN CONVICTUS · MOTTAGNING 3 INFEKTION DANDERYDS SJUKHUS

ACTING UP
"I Have AIDS. Please Hug Me"

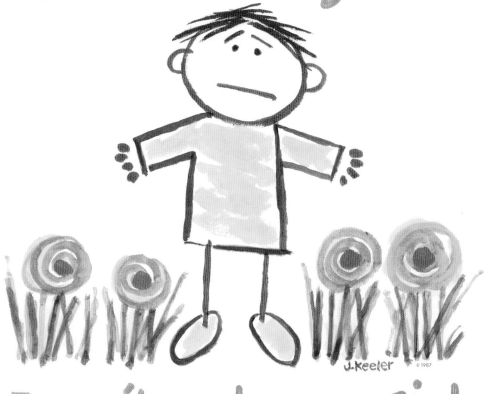

"I Have AIDS. Please Hug Me," 1987
Tiburon, California, U.S.A.
Creator: Center for Attitudinal Healing
Designer: Jack Keeler
38 x 28 cm
AP183

AIDS HOT LINE FOR KIDS
CENTER FOR ATTITUDINAL HEALING
19 MAIN ST., TIBURON, CA 94920, (415) 435-5022

Visual AIDS was founded in 1988 to address the loss to AIDS of those in the arts community and to bring the power of art and the creativity of artists to activism. In 1991, the Visual AIDS Artists' Caucus created the Red Ribbon, which became the most lasting and well-known symbol of AIDS activism. In 1992, the organization began commissioning artists to create black-and-white 8.5 x 11-inch activist "broadsheets" that could be distributed free to the public. This poster is one that John Giorno created in 1993. The size and color scheme had a specific purpose—we wanted it to be easily photocopied by anyone, so that it could be shared with the maximum number of people. An irony of the historicizing of the AIDS activist movement is that broadsheets like this have become part of archival collections and often hang framed on museum walls, taking artworks that were meant to be shared with everyone and activated in public spaces, and instead making them precious and perhaps unattainable to most. Therefore, it is thrilling to us when these pieces can be reactivated. In 2018, the performer Morgan Bassichis chose to activate this particular broadsheet as part of the Whitney Museum of American Art's exhibition

An Incomplete History of Protest: Selections from the Whitney's Collection, 1940–2017. In a Study Session on March 9, 2018, Morgan distributed photocopies of this work, along with its companion piece, and led an assembled audience in chanting and singing the words together. Part of the power of these pieces is that the poignancy continues to ring true today and relates to the human experience both within the AIDS pandemic and beyond it. For our thirtieth anniversary, and inspired in part by Morgan's performance, Visual AIDS reprinted the broadsheet artwork on tote bags so that a new generation can share and experience Giorno's work.

Esther McGowan

Esther McGowan is executive director of the nonprofit arts organization Visual AIDS.

"The World Is Getting Empty of...," 1993
Series: *Day without Art*
Creator: Visual AIDS
Designer: John Giorno
28 x 22 cm
AP1289

THE WORLD IS GETTING EMPTY OF EVERYONE I KNOW ONE BY ONE IN EVERY DIRECTION THEY ARE LEAVING THIS WORLD FOR SOME PEOPLE EVERYONE THEY KNOW HAS DIED

JOHN GIORNO for VISUAL AIDS • NEW YORK • DAY WITHOUT ART • 1993

Funded in part by the Lannan Foundation and the Andy Warhol Foundation for the Visual Arts Inc. © 1993 John Giorno

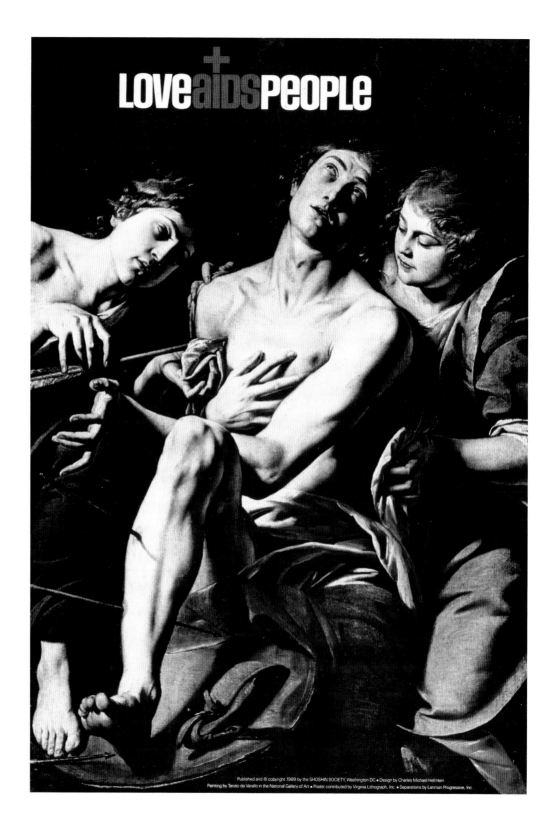

"Love AIDS People," 1988
District of Columbia, U.S.A.
Creator: Shoshin Society
Painting: Tanzio da Varallo
62 x 42 cm
AP564

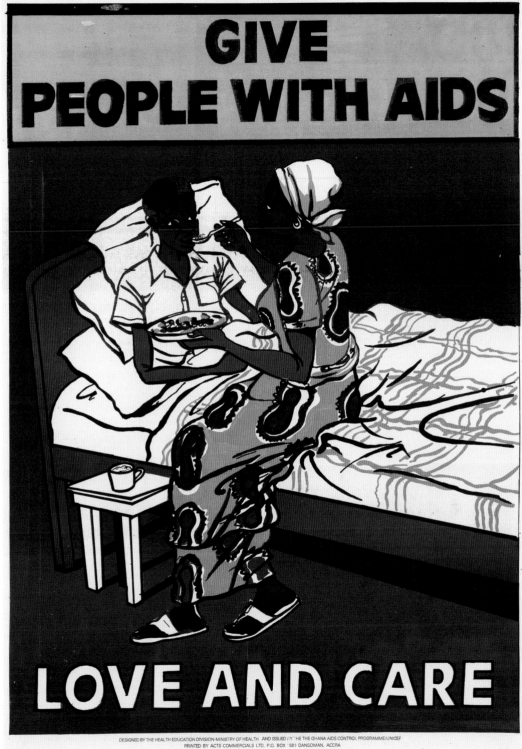

"Give People with AIDS Love and Care,"
n.d.
Accra, Ghana
Creator: National AIDS/STD
Control Programme
62 x 44 cm
AP3436

This poster invokes revolution and resistance, reminiscent of the iconic Medu Art Ensemble. The tricolor palette, here in black, red, and white, and the manipulation of design principles to demonstrate social realities, worldviews, and complex continental relationships, have become somewhat of a tradition in social justice in southern Africa. Whereas the Medu works were produced by exiled cultural workers calling the community to resistance against apartheid, this poster calls for unity and solidarity against the presence of an oppressive pandemic.

Although the artwork is doubly situated, first by the shape of the continent, and second by a cultural marker in the form of a mask, the drift towards greater inclusivity—a trait of many African discourses—can be read from the inclusive pronouns used in the slogan, the collapse of continental borders in definitions of community, the representation of continental kinship, and the implied elevation of agency among civil society.

The central graphic is tiled with profiles of faces and foregrounded by a vigil, represented by a hand holding a candle against a red ribbon. One can see the symbolic use of formal elements and design principles in the highly graphic application of space as a conceptual and emotive element. The negative of one figure is activated and informs the definition of the following figure in succession. One is not implored to read the ascending staccato of silhouettes as literal demographic descriptors such as race, age, gender, or nationality. Instead, this poster makes it possible that the positive and negative spaces be read metaphorically to represent different serostatuses, in an allegory of unity and interdependence among those affected and those infected.

Thus, this poster garners not only the formal elements from the resistance print history of South Africa, but also capitalizes on the visual language that had become synonymous with unity and social mobilization under previous struggles from this region. From its messaging through to its execution, the poster echoes unity and solidarity in many nuanced and interesting ways.

MC Roodt

MC Roodt is arts projects leader at the William Humphreys Art Gallery, an agency of the Department of Arts and Culture, South Africa, and chair for arts and health at the Public Health Association of South Africa.

"Africa We Care. We Can Make a Difference," n.d.
South Africa
Creator: Gauteng AIDS Programme
Designer: Fanela Mashinini
85 x 60 cm
AP3565

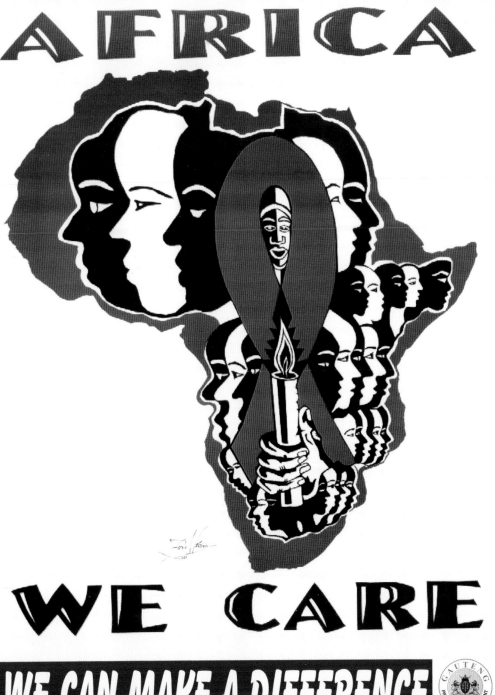

AFRICA

WE CARE

WE CAN MAKE A DIFFERENCE

Gauteng AIDS
Programme

"Caring for People with AIDS," 1992
Series: *Everybody's Business*
Australia
Creator: Commonwealth Department
of Health, Housing and
Community Services
Designer: Bronwyn Bancroft
89 x 61 cm
AP3252

The image, "Final Moments" (1990), was taken by Therese Frare the spring that David Kirby died of complications related to AIDS. Months after, the picture was published in *LIFE* magazine, iconically retitled "The Face of AIDS." Two years later, it was used for what became an infamous Benetton clothing ad, even more powerfully titled "La Pieta." The photograph provides an important and familiar narrative—a frail young man, dying needlessly before his time. And in that, the picture also contains details and absences that speak to stories and dynamics of the ongoing AIDS crisis largely untold, teetering on the precipice of being lost.

The hand on David's wrist belongs to his caregiver, Peta, who, the day the photo was taken, invited Therese, a photography student at the time doing a project on AIDS, to follow as Peta did rounds at the hospice. Therese stayed in the hallway as Peta went in to check on David, a friend, who was near his final days. Therese had met David once before, and he had given her his permission to be photographed.

As Peta visited with David, David's mother invited Therese into the room, asking her to take photos of what could be their last moments all together. On Therese's contact sheets from that day, Peta's whole body can be seen: tall, with long hair pulled back, wearing a black leather jacket. In Peta we meet a caregiver from the Pine Ridge Indian Reservation living with HIV, who, as Therese recalls, "rode the line between genders."

After David died, the Kirbys made a commitment to care for Peta as death approached, and Therese continued to photograph.

Let Peta's wrist—and spirit—encourage viewers to look beyond the poster frame, searching for the stories untold, and the context needed to better understand the history and ongoingness of HIV/AIDS.

Theodore (Ted) Kerr

Theodore (Ted) Kerr is a New York-based writer and a founding member of the collective What Would an HIV Doula Do?

[The Death of David Kirby], 1992
New York, New York, U.S.A.
Creator: United Colors of Benetton
Designers: Tibor Kalman and
Oliviero Toscani with photograph by
Therese Frare
38 x 58 cm
AP8090

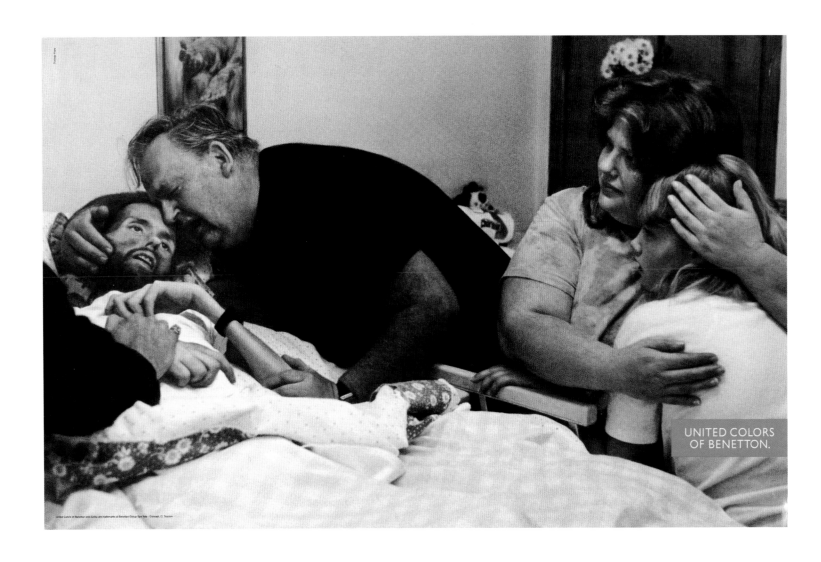

91

Den røde sløyfen symboliserer solidaritet med mennesker som lever med hiv og aids, og er en påminnelse om sikrere sex.

HELSEUTVALGET
FOR · HOMOFILE

"The Red Ribbon Symbolizes Solidarity
with People Living with HIV and AIDS and
Is a Reminder to Have Safer Sex"
(translated from Norwegian), 1995
Oslo, Norway
Creator: Helseutvalget for homofile
60 x 42 cm
AP3991

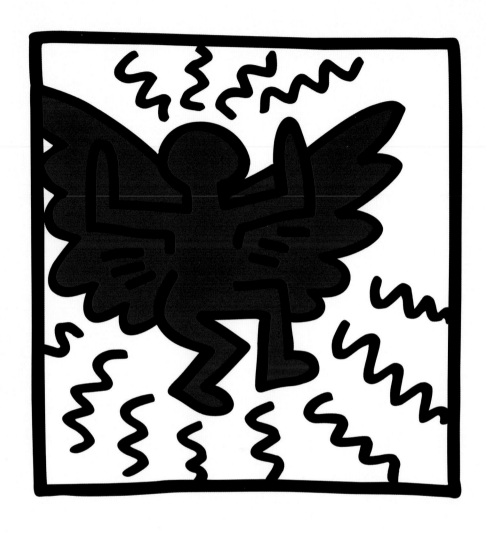

KEITH HARING
The Keith Haring Altarpiece: An AIDS Memorial Chapel Project
Grace Cathedral, San Francisco

"The Keith Haring Altarpiece: An AIDS
Memorial Chapel Project," n.d.
San Francisco, California, U.S.A.
Creator: The McGaw Foundation
Benefitting AIDS Charities
Designer: Keith Haring
92 x 62 cm
AP5213

As a retired ophthalmologist who was in active practice during the very deadly and frightening early years of the AIDS epidemic in the U.S., I continue to be shaken by this poster. In the early to mid-1980s, when the number of AIDS cases began exploding, especially in the gay community, the scientific community was just starting to understand the details about the disease's contagion. Many people, including medical professionals, were afraid of even casual contact with infected persons. It was at that time that I began seeing AIDS patients with severe and often blinding inflammation of the retina (retinitis). Because some of my colleagues were reticent to see these patients, and because I was known to be gay, many of these young men with eye disease were sent to me by local doctors who were just learning to be "AIDS specialists."

It soon became very apparent that the fear of contagion with casual contact was completely unfounded. Shortly thereafter we learned that this retinitis was being caused by a virus, cytomegalovirus, which, although very widespread and benign in the general population, is devastating, frequently blinding, and extremely difficult to treat in the immune-compromised AIDS patient. Sadly, I saw very many wonderful young men become desperately ill, blind, and eventually die of this horrible disease.

Although the AIDS epidemic is still a major worldwide public health problem, it is very encouraging to see the enormous progress that has been made in understanding and treating this deadly disease. For those living in countries with affordable access to good health care, the morbidity and longevity of persons with AIDS has remarkably improved. Indeed, vaccines that could potentially end the epidemic seem to be very much within reach. Nevertheless, until that day, AIDS prevention largely relies on education, and the AIDS poster remains a very relevant educational tool.

Dr. Joseph N. Lambert

Dr. Joseph N. Lambert is an ophthalmologist in Irvine, California.

"AIDS Causes Blindness," n.d.
Boston, Massachusetts, U.S.A.
Creator: AIDS Action Committee of Massachusetts
56 x 43 cm
AP817

AIDS causes blindness.

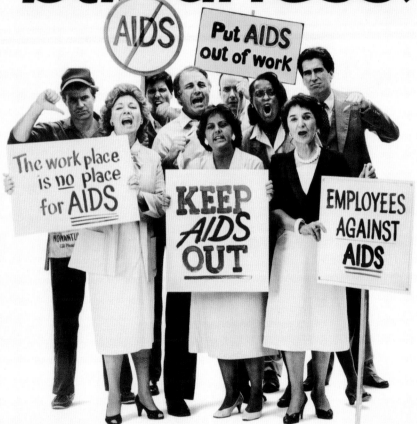

People with AIDS know there's a chance they'll lose their sight. But that's no reason for the people around them to lose sight of the fact that AIDS cannot be caught by touching someone. Or by working around them.

Which means the best way to fight AIDS is not with fear and anger, but with compassion and support.

AIDS ACTION
C O M M I T T E E
661 Boylston Street, Boston, MA 02116
1-800-235-2331

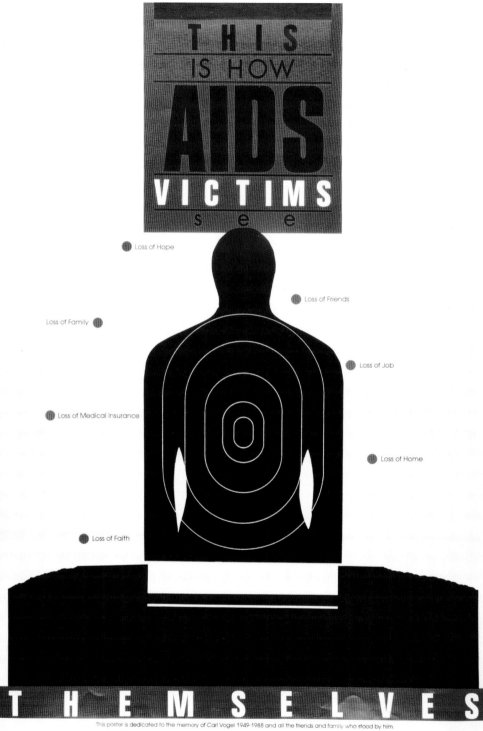

"This Is How AIDS Victims See
Themselves," ca. 1988
Maryland, U.S.A.
Creator: Shoshin Society
Designer: James Thorpe
92 x 61cm
AP6910

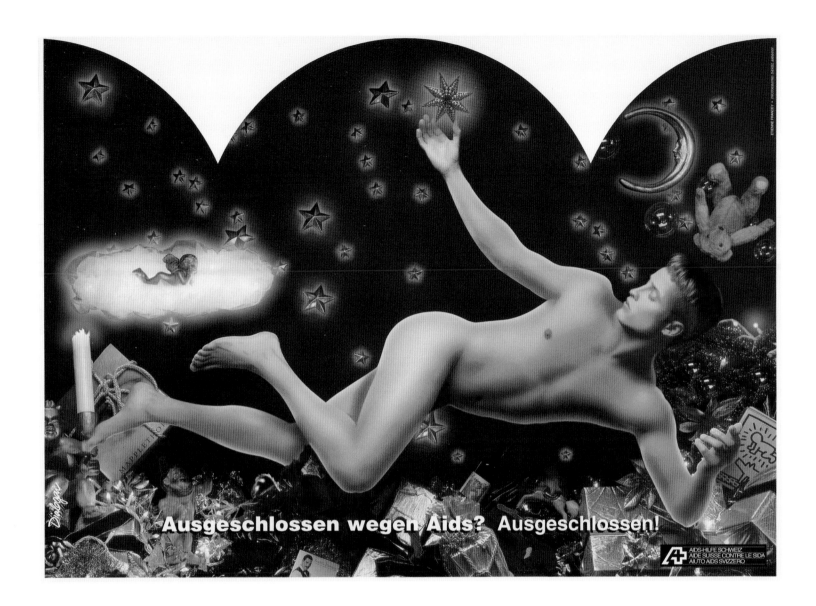

"Excluded Because of AIDS? Locked Out!"
(translated from German), n.d.
Zurich, Switzerland
Creator: AIDS-Hilfe Schweiz
Designer and photographer:
Daniel Ammann
49 x 69 cm
AP5831

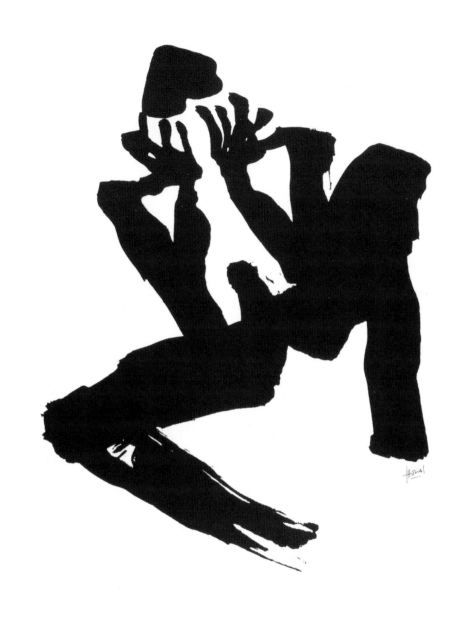

sida
l'isolement n'est pas une solution

parle-nous csam peut t'aider
282.9888

"AIDS. Isolation Is Not a Solution.
Talk to Us. CSAM Can Help You."
(translated from French), n.d.
Montreal, Québec, Canada
Creator: Comité SIDA aide Montréal
60 x 32 cm
AP2458

Of the more than 8,000 posters to choose from in this vast and important collection, I kept going back to this set of four French posters that speak to the horror and pain of stigma relating to HIV/AIDS. Produced by the organization AIDeS, a member of the International AIDS Coalition, these four undated posters are evocative in that they give a not-so-subtle nod to propaganda in the first half of the twentieth century and the dangers of these kinds of imagery and messages. Posters like these have a long historical context, as similar images were used in the 1930s leading up to the rise of the Nazi Party in Germany. They use harsh language, graphic imagery, and blatant stereotypes of the "other," which in this case is the "Sidéen" or the "AIDS sufferer" rather than Jews or other groups targeted during that era. The posters use words such as incompetence, laziness, ineptitude, as well as references to their inability to pay their own way or be responsible for themselves, evoking a sense of fear in the viewer. What is also very interesting about these posters is that they have a mock "wheatpasting" quality and

have been designed to look worn and dated. What also sets them apart are the crisp white "additions" to each poster, reminding the viewer to say, "Non au nouveau ghetto" ("No to the new ghetto") and that we have to commit to non-discrimination of seropositive individuals. They each stand alone as powerful statements about the danger of stigma, but seen together, they are even more compelling. As the curator of record of the AIDS Education Posters collection, I am routinely awed by the strength of the messages and the power of the images. These posters, to me, hold a special place in that they viscerally remind us about the past repeating itself and the importance of treating everyone with kindness and compassion.

Jessica Lacher-Feldman

Jessica Lacher-Feldman is exhibits and special projects manager and curator of the AIDS Education Posters collection at the University of Rochester, River Campus Libraries' Department of Rare Books, Special Collections, and Preservation.

"An AIDS Patient Doesn't Pay His Debts" (translated from French), n.d.
Series: *No to the New Ghetto*
Paris, France
Creator: AIDeS
60 x 40 cm
AP10248

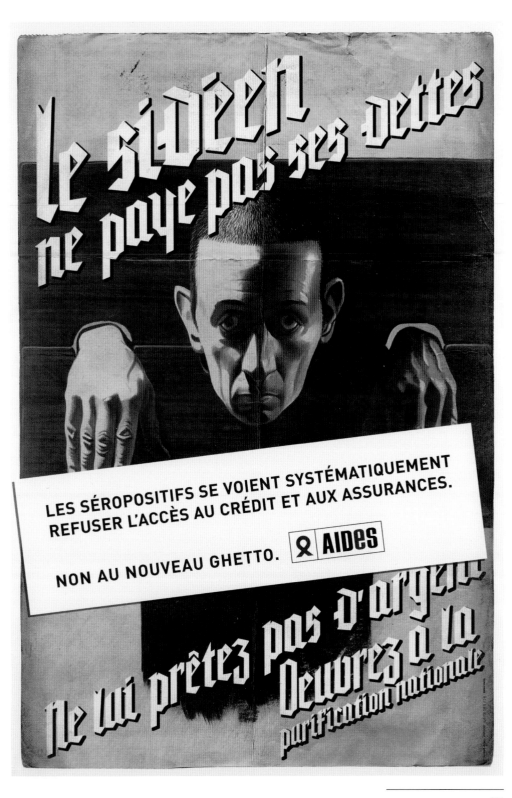

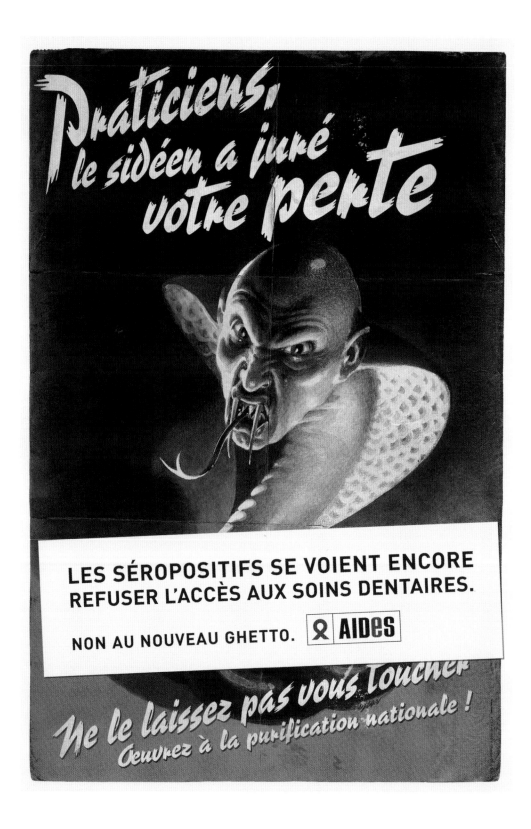

"Practitioners, an AIDS Patient is a Loss
for You" (translated from French), n.d.
Series: *No to the New Ghetto*
Paris, France
Creator: AIDeS
60 x 40 cm
AP10249

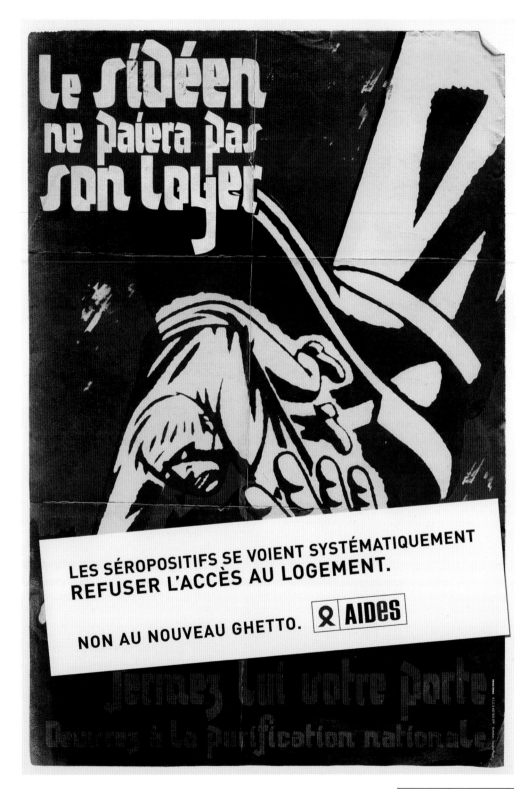

"An AIDS Patient Wouldn't Pay His Rent"
(translated from French), n.d.
Series: *No to the New Ghetto*
Paris, France
Creator: AIDeS
60 x 40 cm
AP10252

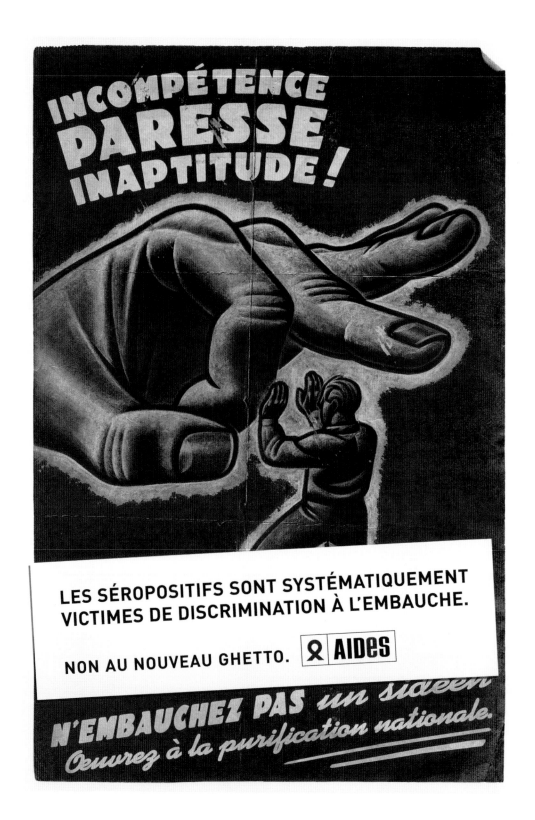

"Incompetence, Laziness, Ineptitude!"
(translated from French), n.d.
Series: *No to the New Ghetto*
Paris, France
Creator: AIDeS
60 x 40 cm
AP10253

"A Homosexual Is Also a Human Being!
Campaign against Anti-Homosexual
Violence" (translated from Portuguese),
n.d.
Brazil
Creator: Centro Baiano Anti-AIDS.
Grupo Gay da Bahia
60 x 40 cm
AP4148

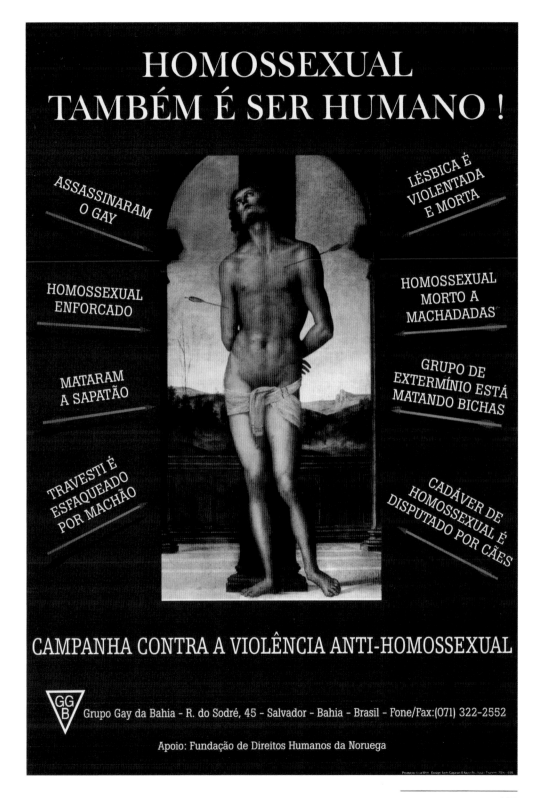

"Care Enough to Love Safely"

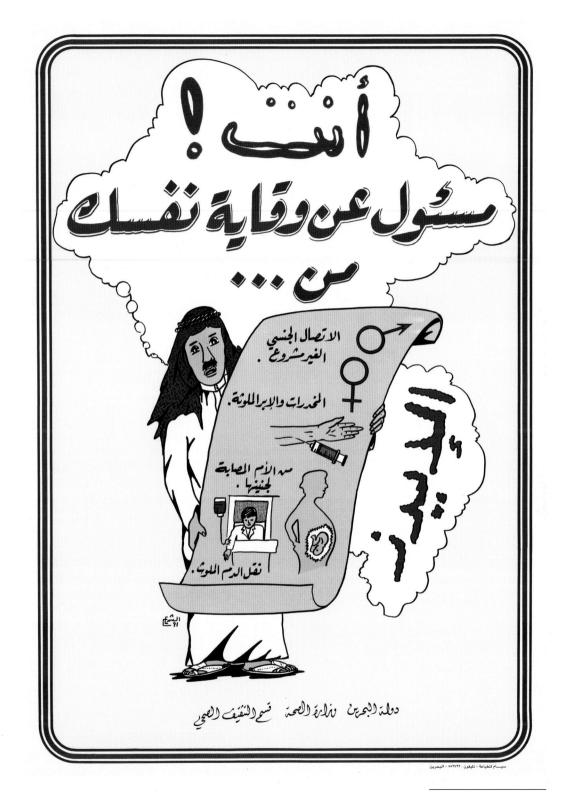

"I Am Responsible for My Actions"
(translated from Arabic), 1991
Bahrain
Creator: Bahrain. Wizarat al-Sihhah
69 x 49 cm
AP3704

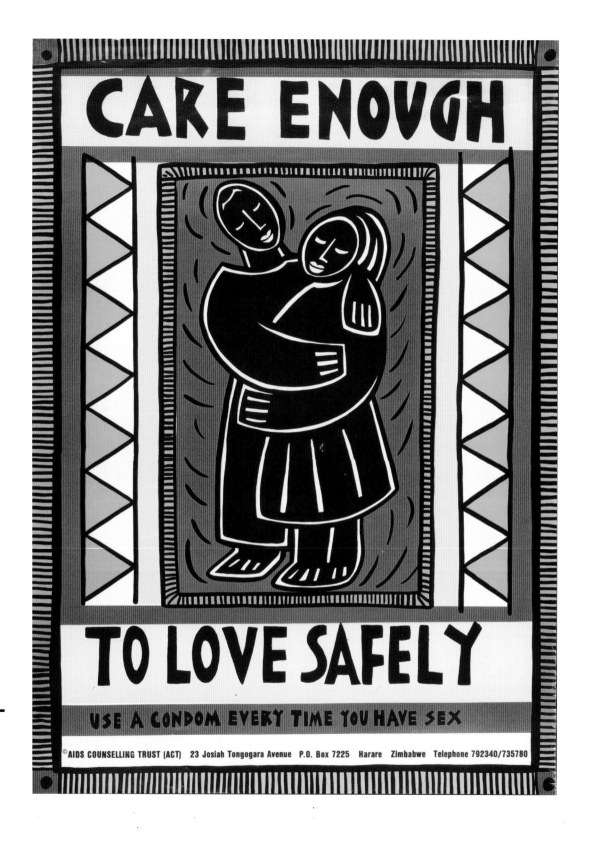

"Care Enough to Love Safely," 1993
Harare, Zimbabwe
Creator: AIDS Counseling Trust
60 x 42 cm
AP3522

"Love Carefully," 1988
Arizona, U.S.A.
Creator: White Mountain Apache Tribe
of the Fort Apache Reservation, Arizona
Health Education Department
56 x 36 cm
AP7017

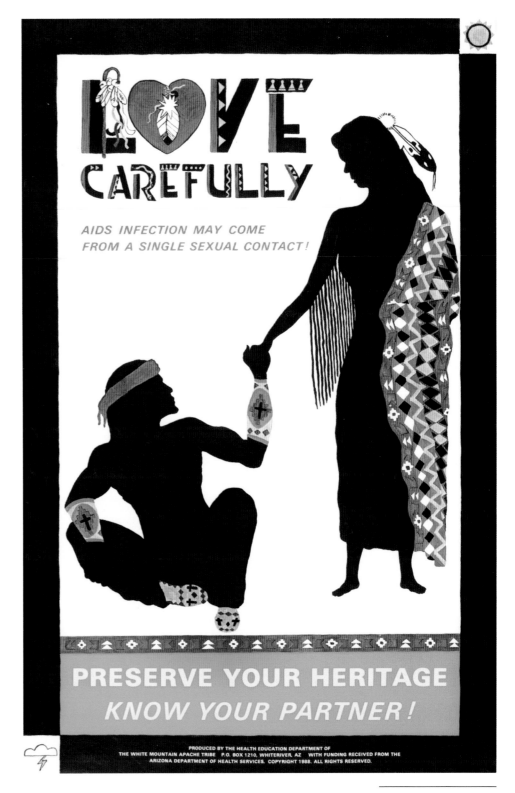

Glede og omsorg

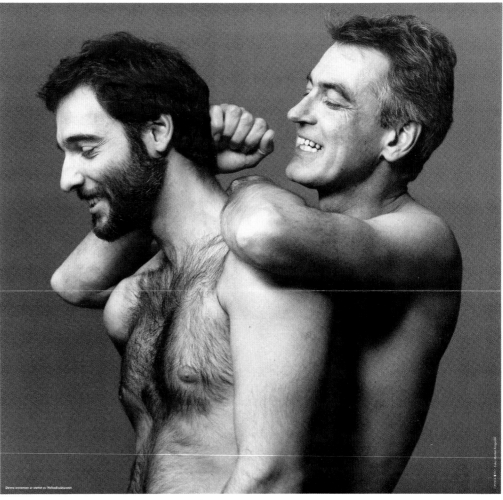

AIDS regnes i dag for en dødelig sykdom, som forårsakes av et virus kalt HIV. Viruset overføres først og fremst gjennom seksuell omgang. Man vet at den største risikogruppen i vår del av verden, er menn som har sex med menn.

Du bør vite at viruset lettest overføres via sæd og blod. Unngå derfor å få i deg noe av dette. Bruker du kondom minsker du risikoen. Det er en rimelig investering for å forebygge AIDS. Husk også at kondomer utsettes for større belastning ved anal-sex. Vannluselige glidekremer og hensynsfullhet bør være en selvfølge.

Du kan selv være bærer av viruset uten å ha symptomer eller bli syk. Derfor bør du regne deg som en potensiell bærer, og være klar over at du *kan* overføre HIV til dine seksualpartnere.

Seksualitet er en naturlig del av livet ditt.
De erotiske følelsene dine skal du ikke stenge inne. Selv om

det er et faktum at også *du* kan rammes av AIDS eller være bærer av viruset, så er det ingen fornuft i at du skal nekte deg en av livets største gaver.

Slike tanker kan bare skape frustrasjon og avstand til de mennesker du er glad i. Det beste hensynet du kan ta til deg selv og andre, er ganske enkelt å tenke over *hva* du gjør *for* du gjør det.

Omsorg øker gleden.
Hvis du begynner å snakke åpent om sex, vil du oppdage at mange tenker som deg. Det er bare ikke like lett for alle å snakke om følelser. Ja, noen tror faktisk at sikrere sex er så kjedelig at det ikke er verd å snakke om – langt mindre å prøve!

Du kan være med på å overbevise andre om at de tar feil. Sikrere sex betyr jo først og fremst å ha større omsorg for hverandre. Slik at ingen får i seg sæd eller blod.

Derfor er kondom alltid en god beskyttelse.
Når du beskytter deg selv, beskytter du også andre. Da viser du at sikrere sex snarere blir en utfordring enn begrensning i leken.

Vil du vite mer om sikrere sex? Da bør du lese brosjyren: «10 helsevettregler for menn som har sex med menn». Ta kontakt med Helseutvalget for homofile, tlf. (02) 36 06 46.

Du kan skrive til oss eller stikke innom, adressen er Øvre Slottsgate 5, p.b. 1305 Vika, 0112 Oslo 1. Vi har også en automatisk telefonsvarer med råd om sikrere sex, tlf. 36 07 30.

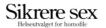
Helseutvalget for homofile

Andre aktuelle adresser: DNF-48, Oslo-region, Boks 1305, Vika, Oslo 1. Telefon 02. 42 08 54. AHF, Boks 5390 Majorstua, 0304 Oslo 3. Telefon: 02. 29 30 51. Oslo Helseråd, Avd. for Tiltak mot AIDS, St. Olavs plass 5, 0165 Oslo 1. Oslo Helseråds informasjonstelefon om AIDS. Telefon 02. 20 65 55.

"Joy and Care. Safer Sex"
(translated from Norwegian), 1986–87
Series: *Jeg er hiv-smittet. Gi meg en klem*
Oslo, Norway
Creator: Helseutvalget for homofile
56 x 44 cm
AP3977

110

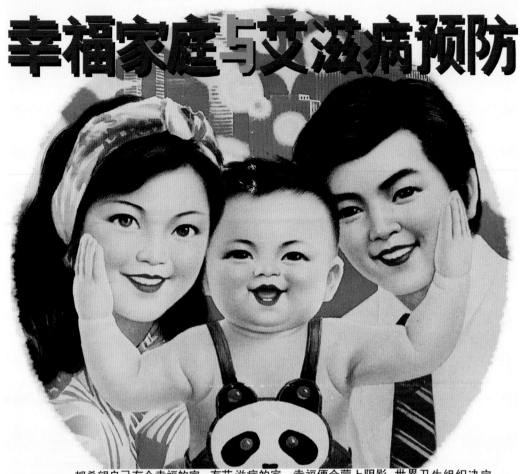

幸福家庭与艾滋病预防

都希望自己有个幸福的家。有艾滋病的家，幸福便会蒙上阴影。世界卫生组织决定
今年艾滋病的主题是："家庭与艾滋病"。社会大家庭预防艾滋病需要每个小家庭作出贡献。

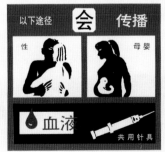

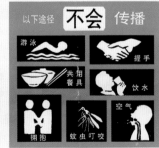

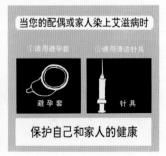

咨询电话：4145711—248、8181788、3132353

云南省卫生厅、 云南省艾滋病防治领导小组办公室

"Happy Family and AIDS Prevention"
(translated from Chinese), n.d.
China
Creator: Chinese Association of STD
and AIDS Control and Prevention
78 x 55 cm
AP5321

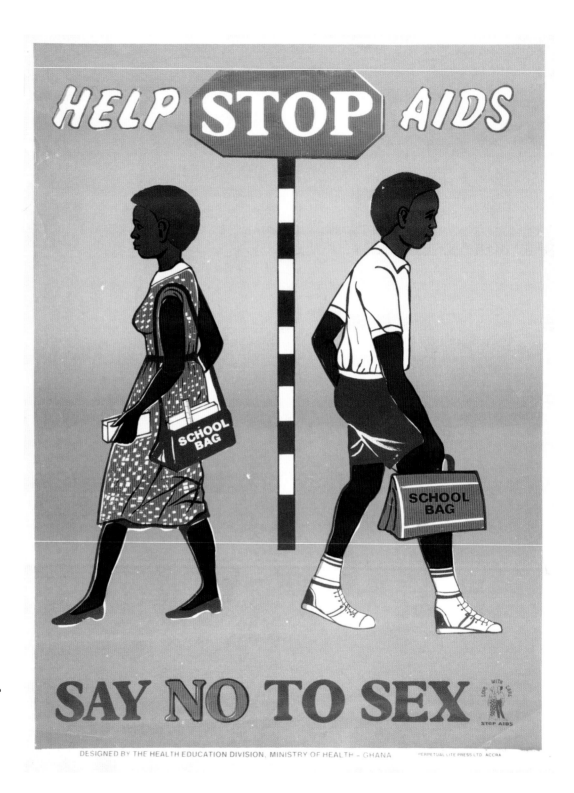

"Help Stop AIDS. Say No to Sex," n.d.
Accra, Ghana
Creator: National AIDS/STD Control
Programme
62 x 45 cm
AP3509

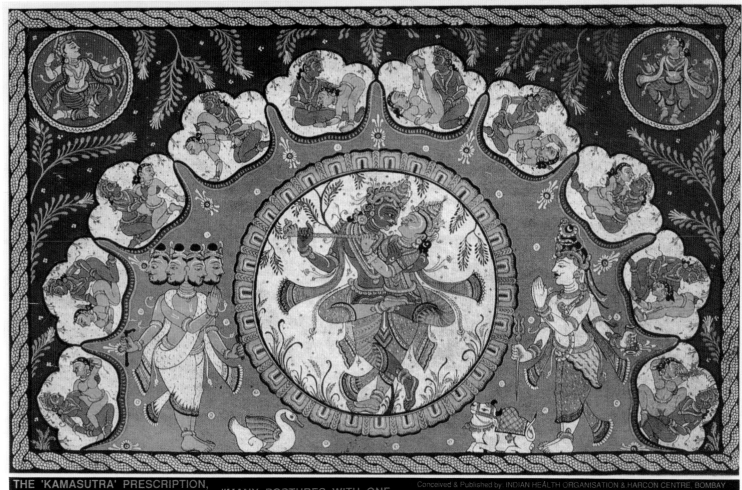

"The 'Kamasutra' Prescription, to Avoid
HIV Infection...'Many Postures with One
Better Than One with Many,'" n.d.
Mumbai, India
Creator: Indian Health Organization
30 x 44 cm
AP3741

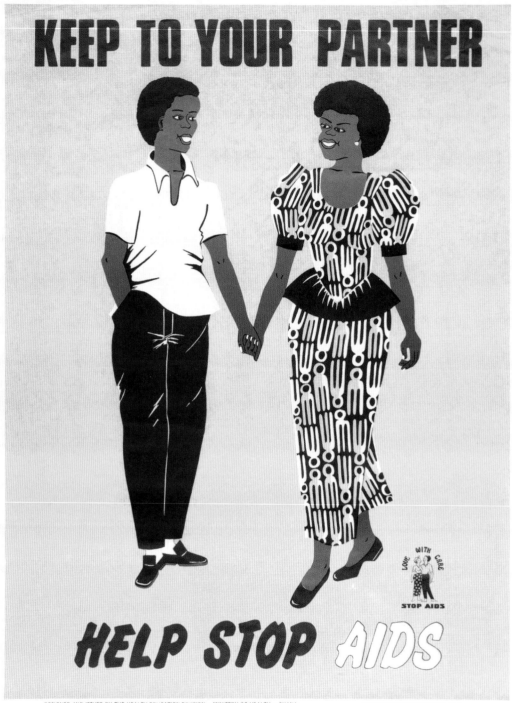

"Keep to Your Partner. Help Stop AIDS,"
n.d.
Accra, Ghana
Creator: Health Education Division
Ministry of Health
61 x 46 cm
AP3510

114

In 2011, HIV-positive performance artist Mikiki and their collaborator Scott Donald made the poster "I Party, I Bareback, I'm Positive, I'm Responsible" for the Toronto-based PosterVirus, an affinity project of the direct-action group AIDS Action Now! As part of the PosterVirus praxis, the poster was plastered up across the streets of Toronto and dispersed online through social media. The poster itself entered the public sphere at a time when there had been a lull in public discussions about HIV. This was just on the cusp of the giant wave of PrEP (Pre-Exposure Prophylaxis) washing over responses to HIV. While widely known by people living with HIV, understandings of "undetectable equalling untransmittable" (U = U) had also not yet gained institutional recognition. As a result, Mikiki's poster acted like a bomb blowing apart institutionalized understandings of people living with HIV as problems to be managed, surveilled, and controlled to assert new claims of sexual agency that were not possible before.

The poster caused public outcry, a firestorm of social media fights, public meetings in various cities across Canada, forcing conversations on choice, condomless sex, drug use, and responsibility. Some saw the message as an attack on past responses, where safer sex was a collective responsibility for community well-being. Others understood the message as staking a claim on a sexual subjectivity in a new post-condom era, aimed at disrupting the ways in which people living with HIV had been denied autonomy and sexual decision-making.

Alexander McClelland

Alexander McClelland, Ph.D., who is living with HIV, is a Banting Postdoctoral Fellow, Department of Criminology at the University of Ottawa.

"I Party, I Bareback, I'm Positive, I'm Responsible," n.d.
Toronto, Ontario, Canada
Creator: AIDS Action Now!
43 x 28 cm
AP13604

I PARTY
I BAREBACK
I'M POSITIVE
I'M RESPONSIBLE

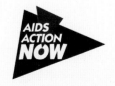

Japan's economy underwent unprecedented growth throughout the 1980s, opening its borders to migrant workers from Southeast Asia in order to meet an increasing demand for labor. Japan is a historically isolationist nation, and this new wave of immigration raised a set of concerns around border control and national identity that framed responses to HIV/AIDS in the country.

The Japanese Foundation for AIDS Prevention (JFAP) was founded in 1987 with support from the Japanese government, after a series of media panics in Japan demanded an official response. These sensationalized reports began in November 1986 with news of a Filipina woman who had tested positive for HIV in the Philippines, and was believed to be working in Japan as a hostess at a strip bar. Nightclubs responded by posting notices declaring "No Filipina dancers," and health officials specifically encouraged men who had slept with foreign women to get tested, quickly cementing a link between foreigners, sex work, and HIV. Shortly after these panics, a bill was passed that enforced mandatory reporting of HIV diagnoses, and gave immigration authorities the right to deny entry to any foreigner who could potentially transmit the virus.[1]

Tacitly acknowledging the widespread practices of extramarital sex and sexual tourism among Japanese salarymen, this poster illustrates the anxieties around sex work and foreigners that characterized the Japanese response during the first decade of the epidemic. Locating the threat of AIDS outside of the island nation of Japan, the poster casts travel as a euphemism for sex with foreigners and posits an image of the nation—the passport—as metaphorical protection from foreign contamination.

The Japanese artist and activist Teiji Furuhashi has cited this poster's xenophobic and heteronormative tone as an impetus for the creation of the AIDS Poster Project in 1992, an organization that produced alternative safer sex campaigns aimed at gay men and lesbians.[2] In 1994, Japan's isolationist AIDS policies came under global scrutiny during the International AIDS Conference in Yokohama, when an American AIDS activist was detained after voluntarily disclosing his HIV status on his immigration card. Though the Japanese government opened its borders to people living with HIV after the incident, sex workers remained banned from entry, and the rhetoric of containment and foreign contamination continued to be a central concern of Japanese AIDS activists throughout the 1990s.

Kyle Croft

Kyle Croft is programs manager at Visual AIDS in New York City

1. Elizabeth Miller, "What's in a Condom? HIV and Sexual Politics in Japan," *Culture, Medicine and Psychiatry* 26 (2002): 1–32.
2. Glenn Sumi, "Activating Art with AIDS: Teiji Furuhashi Tries to Rid Today's Japan of Shame and Ignorance," *Xtra! Toronto's Gay and Lesbian News* (September 29, 1995).

"Have a Nice Trip. But Be Careful of AIDS" (translated from Japanese), 1991
Series: *Sharing the Challenge*
Japan
Creator: Japanese Foundation for AIDS Prevention
84 x 60 cm
AP5337

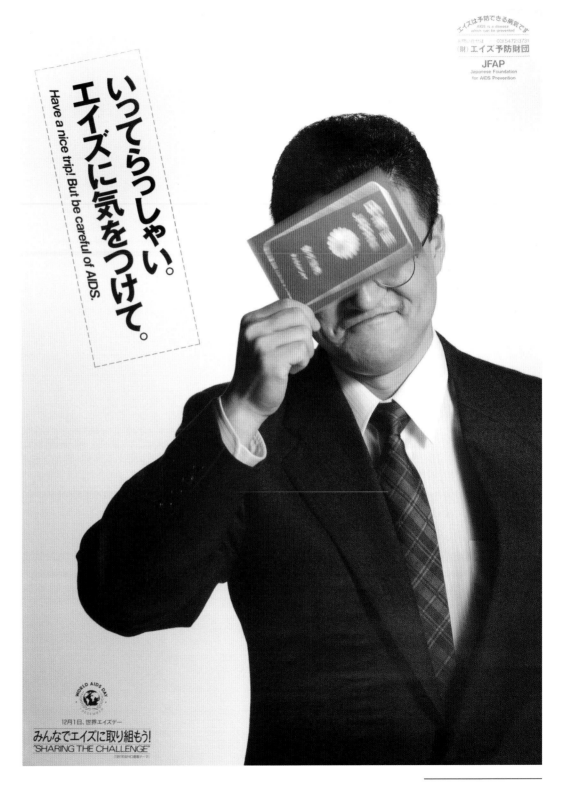

いってらっしゃい。
エイズに気をつけて。

Have a nice trip! But be careful of AIDS.

エイズは予防できる病気です
AIDS is a disease
which can be prevented

お問い合わせは　03(5472)3731
(財) エイズ予防財団
JFAP
Japanese Foundation
for AIDS Prevention

12月1日、世界エイズデー
みんなでエイズに取り組もう！
"SHARING THE CHALLENGE"

"These Go with Everything!"

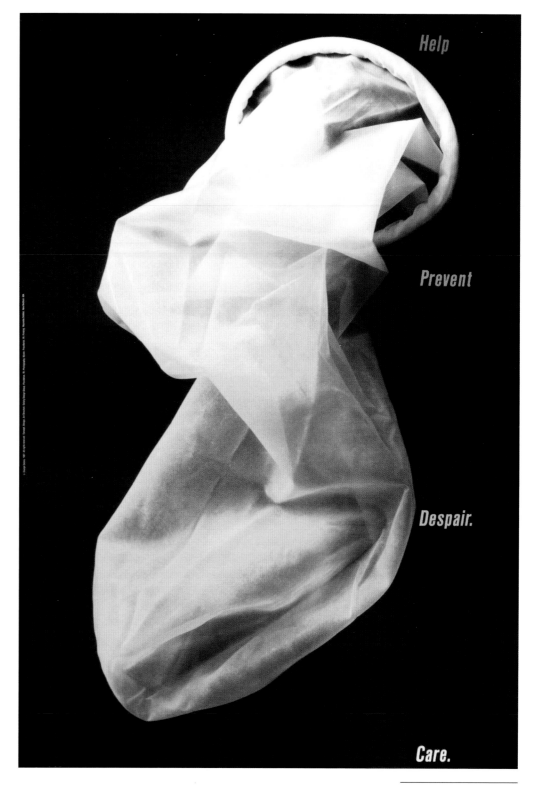

Help

Prevent

Despair.

Care.

"Help Prevent Despair. Care," 1987
Providence, Rhode Island, U.S.A.
Creator: Delany Design Group
92 x 61 cm
AP5271

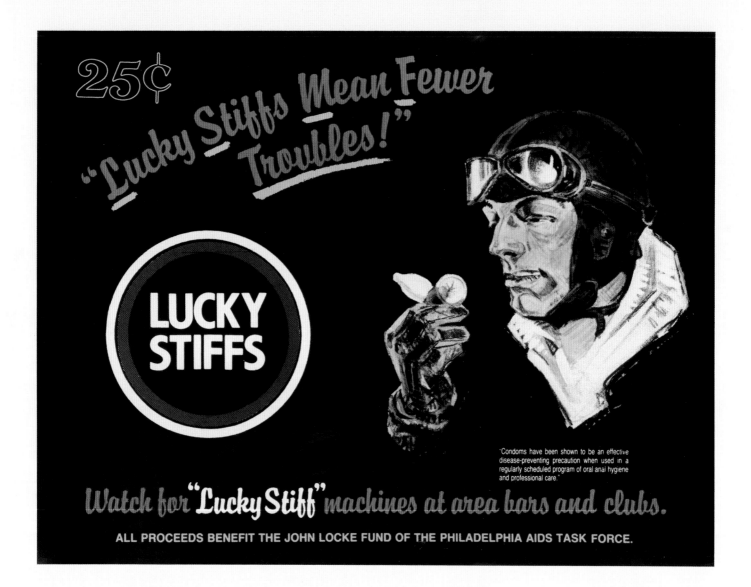

"Lucky Stiffs Mean Fewer Troubles!" n.d.
Philadelphia, Pennsylvania, U.S.A.
Creator: Philadelphia AIDS Task force
41 x 51 cm
AP1542

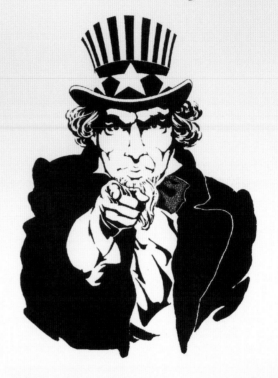

If you are sexually active...

I WANT YOU
TO USE CONDOMS

Stop AIDS. Do It Now.

A public service message of the Do It Now Foundation • Box 27568 • Tempe, AZ 85285 • (602) 491-0393

"If You Are Sexually Active...
I Want You to Use Condoms," 1993
Tempe, Arizona, U.S.A.
Creator: Do It Now Foundation
Illustration inspired by James
Montgomery Flagg
42 x 26 cm
AP33

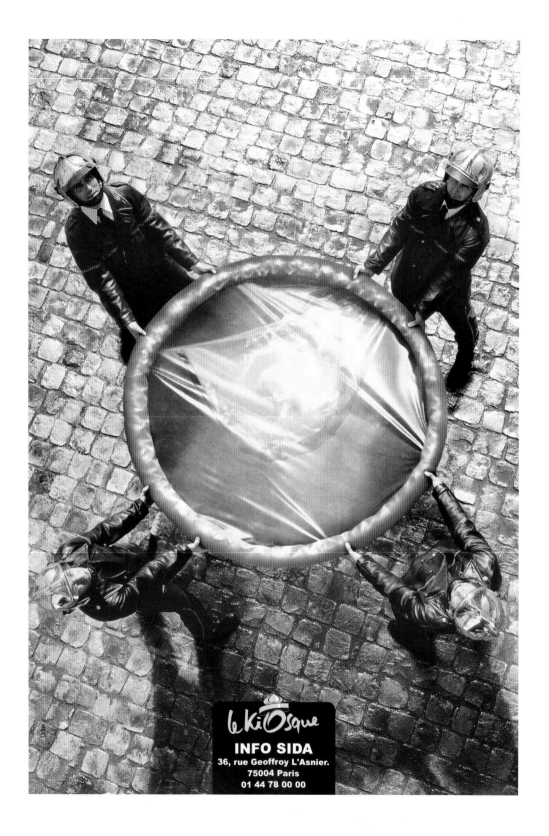

"The Stand" (translated from French), n.d.
Paris, France
Creator: Kiosque
60 x 40 cm
AP6463

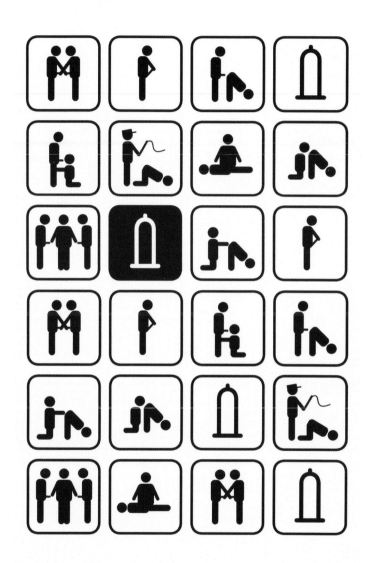

MANNENSEKS.BE
de gay site van sensoa

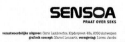

SENSOA
PRAAT OVER SEKS

verantwoordelijke uitgever: Chris Lambrechts, Kipdorpvest 48a, 2000 Antwerpen
grafisch concept: Marcel Lennartz, vormgeving: Lieven Jacobs

"Mannenseks.Be—The Gay Site of
SENSOA" (translated from Dutch), n.d.
Series: *SENSOA pictograms*
Antwerp, Belgium
Creator: SENSOA
Designer: Lieven Jacobs
Graphic Concept: Marcel Lennartz
63 x 30 cm
AP11080_01

"Prevention of AIDS," 1992
Series: *Everybody's Business*
Australia
Creator: Commonwealth Department of
Health, Housing, Local Government and
Community Services
Designer: Bronwyn Bancroft
89 x 61 cm
AP3253

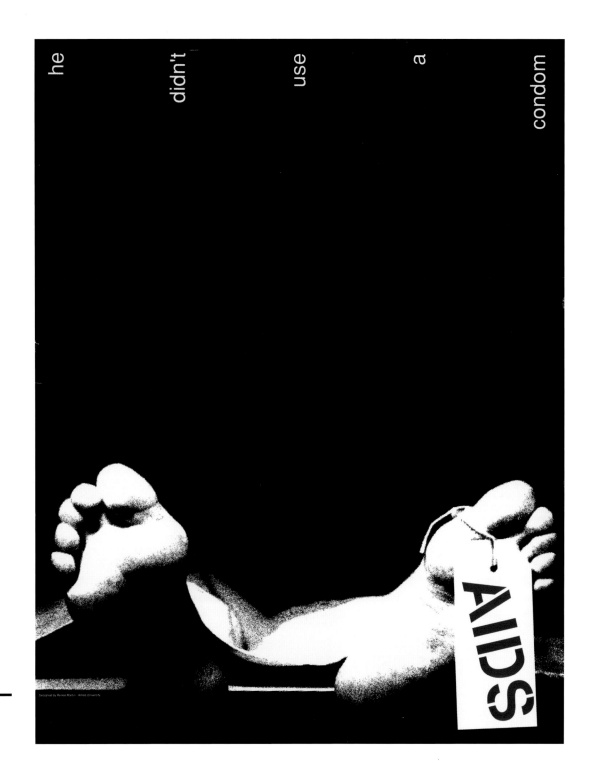

"He Didn't Use a Condom. AIDS," n.d.
Alfred, New York, U.S.A.
Creator: Alfred University
Designer: Renee Martin
56 x 43 cm
AP1117

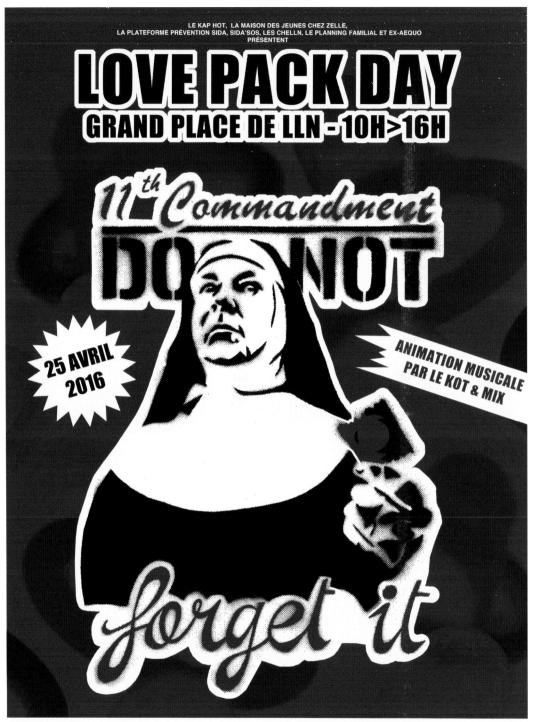

"11th Commandment. Do Not Forget It,"
2016
Belgium
Creator: Kap Hot
59 x 42 cm
AP13709

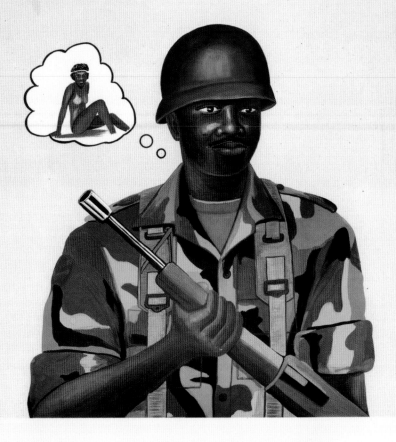

"Combat Readiness. Condom Readiness,"
1993
Accra, Ghana
Creator: National AIDS/STD
Control Programme
Designer: Apple Pie Publicity
64 x 46 cm
AP3503

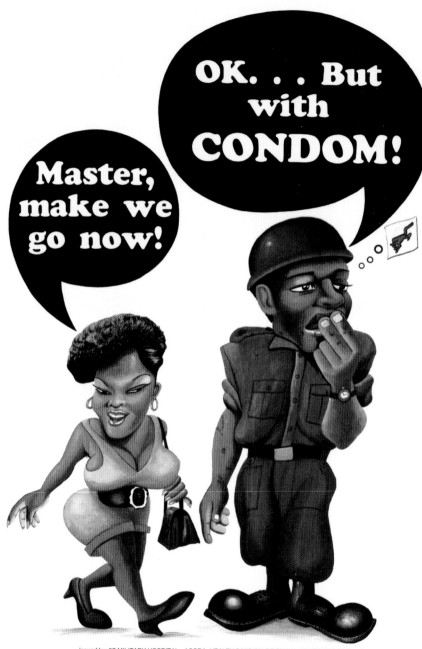

"Master, Make We Go Now!
OK... But with Condom!" n.d.
Accra, Ghana
Creator: National AIDS/STD
Control Programme
Designer: Apple Pie Publicity
28 x 22 cm
AP5988

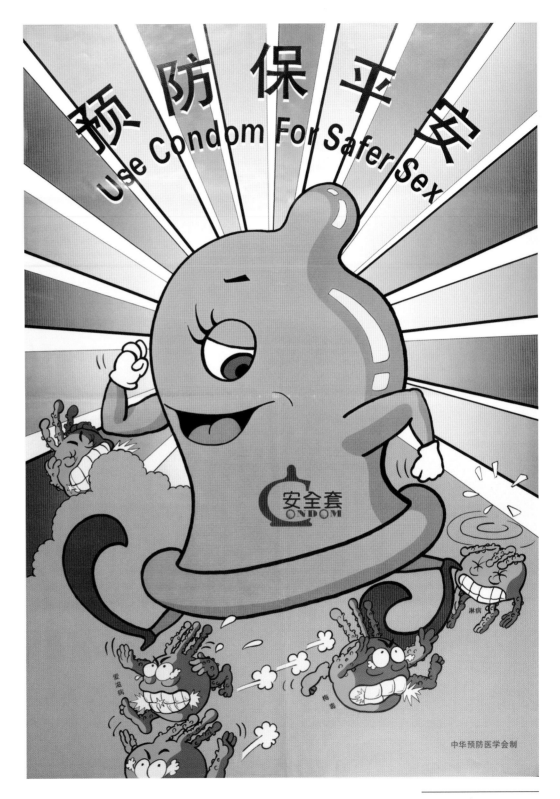

"Use Condom for Safer Sex," n.d.
Hong Kong
Creator: Hong Kong Department of
Health, AIDS Unit
77 x 51 cm
AP5355

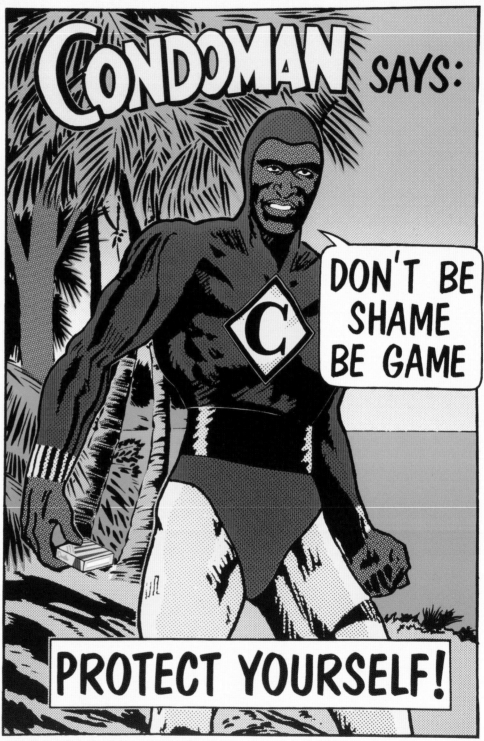

"Condoman Says: Don't Be Shame,
Be Game. Protect Yourself!" 1991
Woden, Australia
Creator: Australia Department of Health,
Housing and Community Services
42 x 28 cm
AP3264

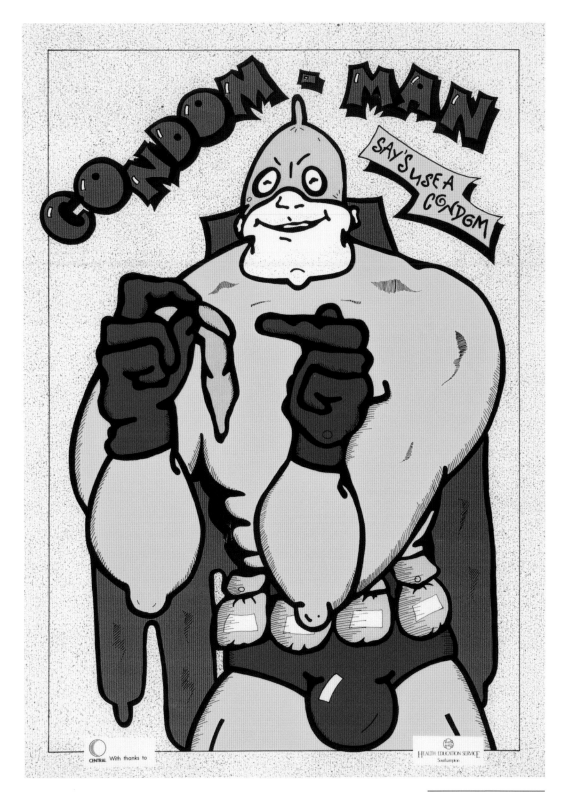

"Condom-Man Say's [*sic*] Use a Condom,"
n.d.
England, UK
Creator: Health Education Service
Southampton
42 x 30 cm
AP6172

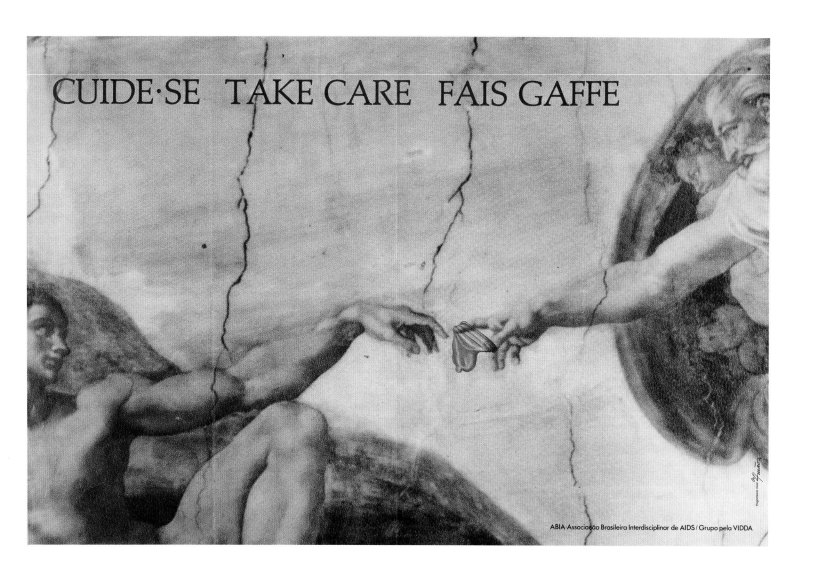

CUIDE·SE TAKE CARE FAIS GAFFE

ABIA·Associação Brasileira Interdisciplinar de AIDS / Grupo pela VIDDA

"Take Care," n.d.
Rio de Janeiro, Brazil
Creator: ABIA—Associação Brasileira
Interdisciplinar de AIDS/Grupo
pela Vidda
Fresco: Michelangelo Buonarroti
62.5 x 91.5 cm
AP10334_01

THE ART OF LIVING

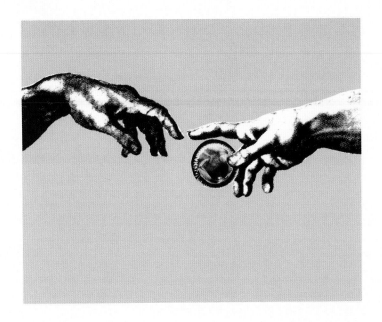

"The Art of Living," n.d.
Series: *The Art of Living*
Los Angeles, California, U.S.A.
Creator: Stop AIDS Los Angeles, a division of the Gay and Lesbian Community Services Center
Designers: Erik A. Armstrong, Charles C. Oh, Manuela Zaretti
Image: Michelangelo Buonarroti
57 x 45 cm
AP146

"The Art of Living" is a safer sex campaign presented by STOP AIDS Los Angeles which is a division of the Gay and Lesbian Community Services Center and is funded by the State of California and the County of Los Angeles.   Poster design by: Erik A. Armstrong, Charles C. Oh & Manuela Zaretti

True Love.

If you care for each other, protect each other. Use a latex condom every time.

It's not 100% protection against AIDS—only doing without sex and IV drugs entirely does that—but it cuts your risk considerably. For more information, call the AIDS hotline in Northern California at 1-800-367-2437, or in Southern California at 1-800-922-2437.

AIDS.
It's Up To You.
State of California AIDS Education Campaign

"True Love," 1994
Series: *AIDS: It's Up to You*
Santa Cruz, California, U.S.A.
Creator: State of California
AIDS Education Campaign
64 x 49 cm
AP409

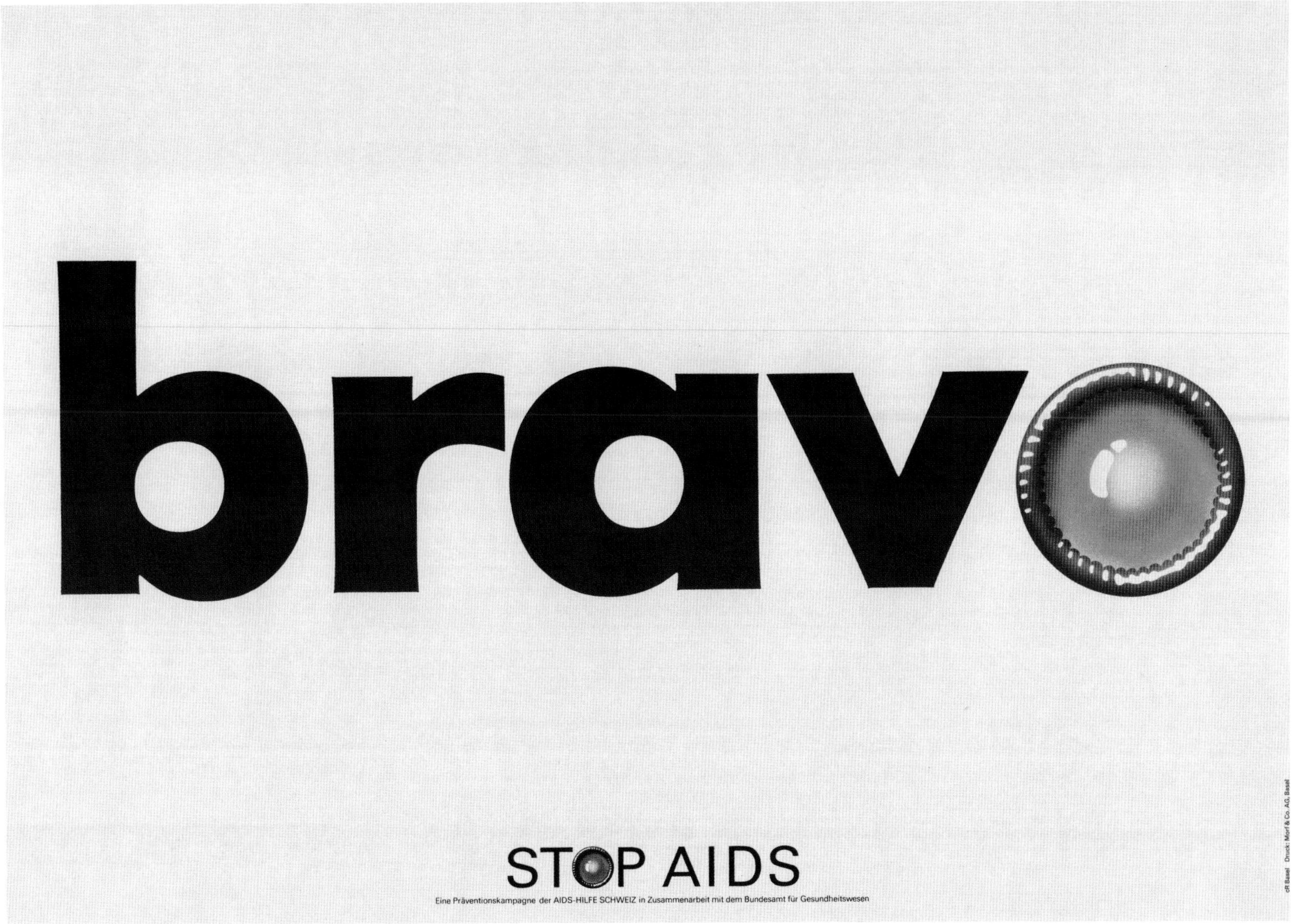
bravo
STOP AIDS
Eine Präventionskampagne der AIDS-HILFE SCHWEIZ in Zusammenarbeit mit dem Bundesamt für Gesundheitswesen
cR Basel Druck: Morf & Co. AG, Basel

"Bravo: Stop AIDS," 1988
Zurich, Switzerland
Creator: AIDS-Hilfe Schweiz
Designer: cR Basel
42 x 60 cm
AP5841

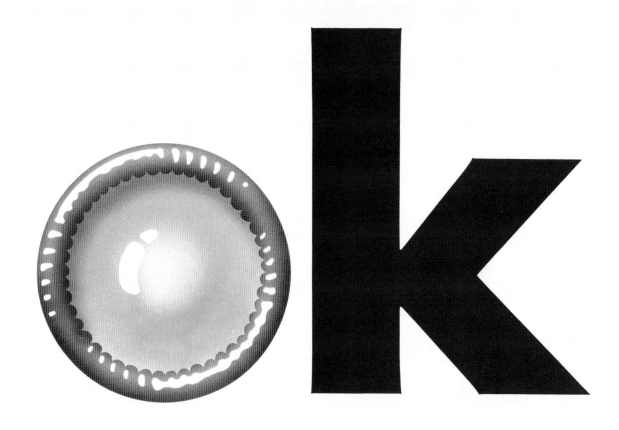

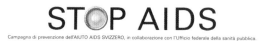

STOP AIDS

Campagna di prevenzione dell'AIUTO AIDS SVIZZERO, in collaborazione con l'Ufficio federale della sanità pubblica.

"OK: Stop AIDS," 1988
Zurich, Switzerland
Creator: AIDS-Hilfe Schweiz
Designer: cR Basel
42 x 60 cm
AP5839

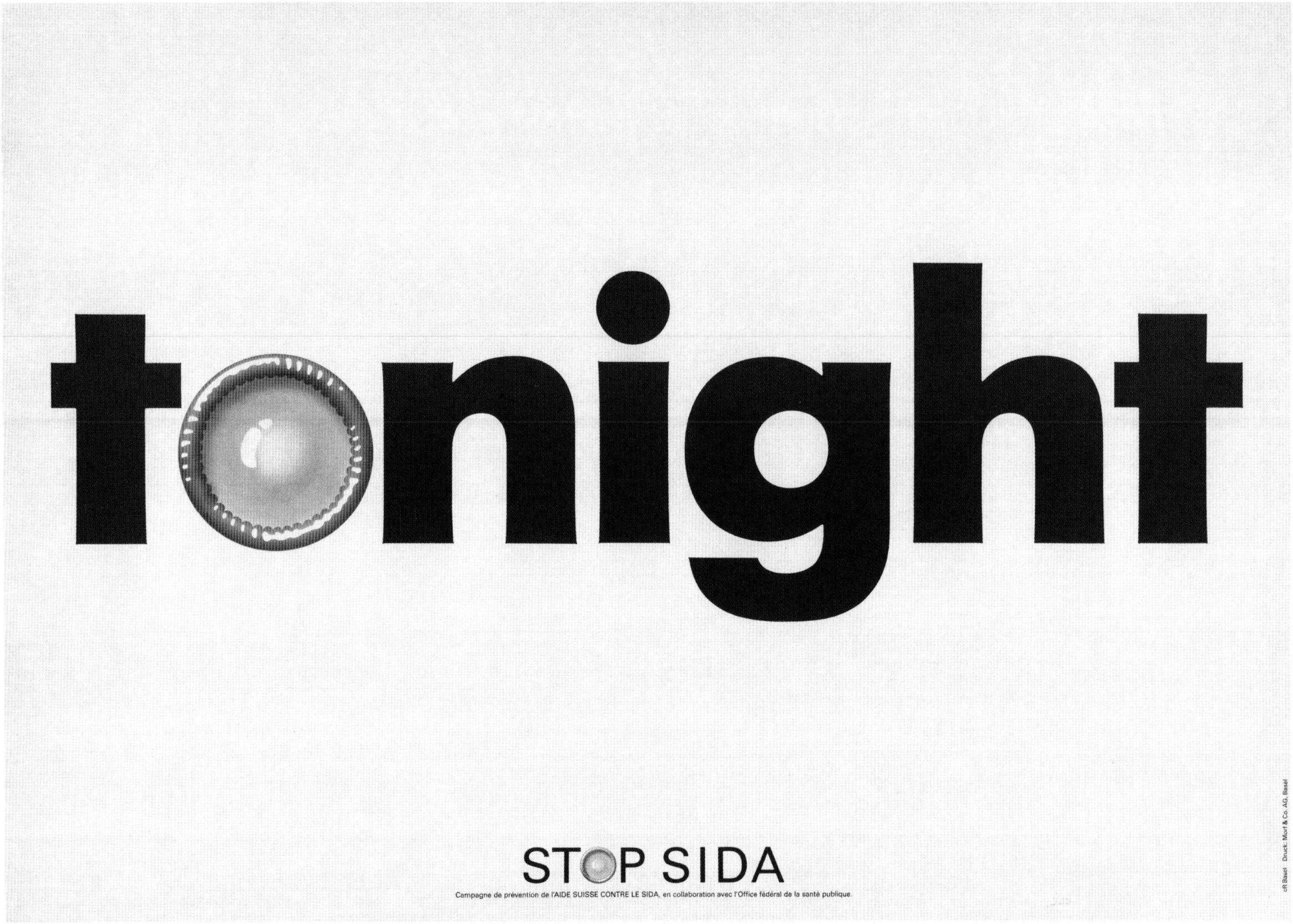

tonight
STOP SIDA
Campagne de prévention de l'AIDE SUISSE CONTRE LE SIDA, en collaboration avec l'Office fédéral de la santé publique.
cR Basel Druck: Mort & Co. AG, Basel

"Tonight: Stop SIDA," 1988
Zurich, Switzerland
Creator: AIDS-Hilfe Schweiz
Designer: cR Basel
42 x 60 cm
AP5840

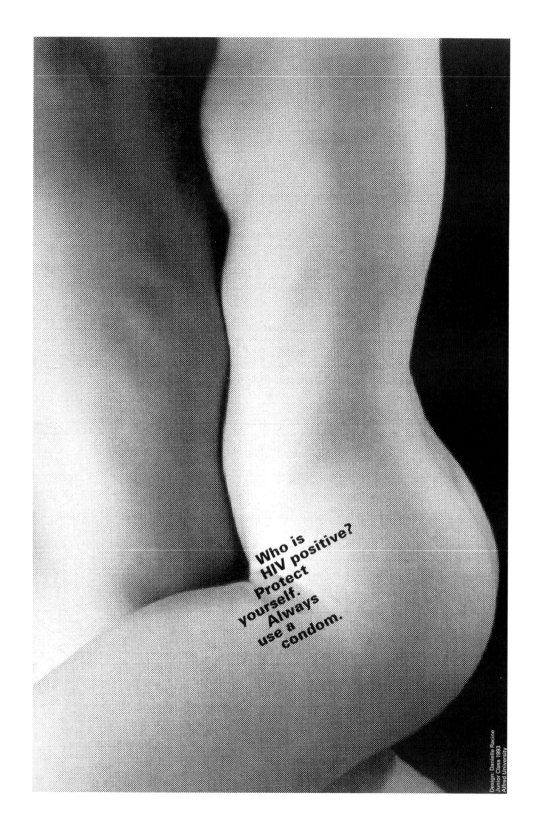

Who is
HIV positive?
Protect
yourself.
Always
use a
condom.

Design: Danielle Racine
Junior Class 1993
Alfred University

"Who Is HIV Positive? Protect Yourself.
Always Use a Condom," 1993
Alfred, New York, U.S.A.
Creator: Alfred University
Designer: Danielle Racine
43 x 28 cm
AP1105

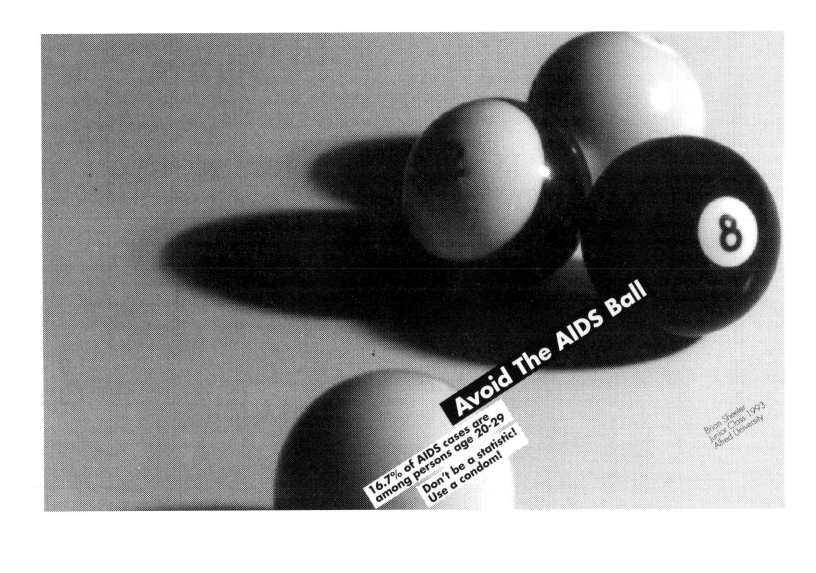

Avoid The AIDS Ball

16.7% of AIDS cases are among persons age 20-29

Don't be a statistic! Use a condom!

Brian Sheeler
Junior Class 1993
Alfred University

"Avoid the AIDS Ball," 1993
Alfred, New York, U.S.A.
Creator: Alfred University
Designer: Brian Sheeler
28 x 43 cm
AP1106

"Do You Want to Screw? AIDS. Think
before You Act. Protect Yourself," 1993
Alfred, New York, U.S.A.
Creator: Alfred University
Designer: Kristie L. Atwood
43 x 28 cm
AP1108

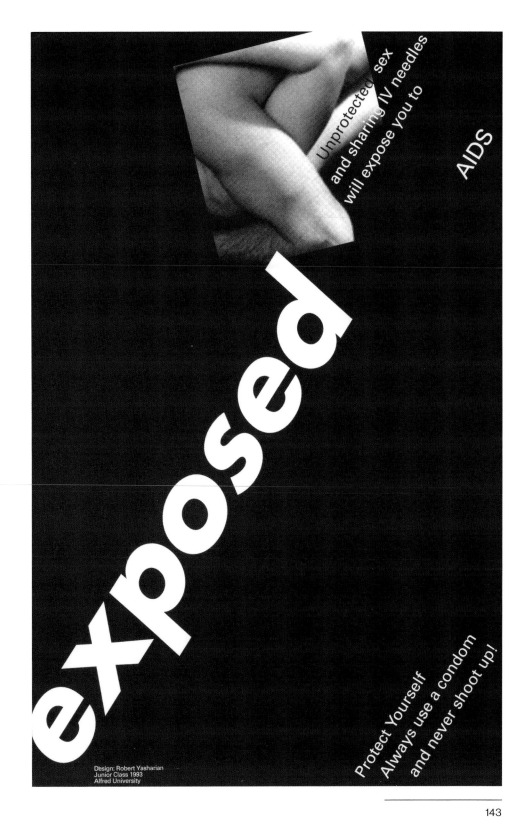

"Exposed. Protect Yourself. Always Use a
Condom and Never Shoot Up!" 1993
Alfred, New York, U.S.A.
Creator: Alfred University
Designer: Robert Yasharian
43 x 28 cm
AP1107

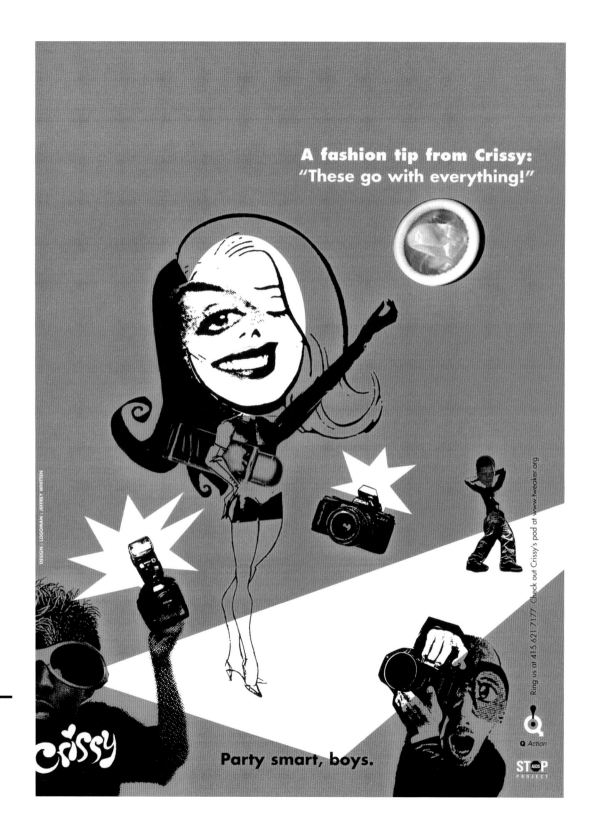

"A Fashion Tip from Crissy:
'These Go with Everything!'" n.d.
San Francisco, California, U.S.A.
Creator: Stop AIDS Project
31 x 22 cm
AP356

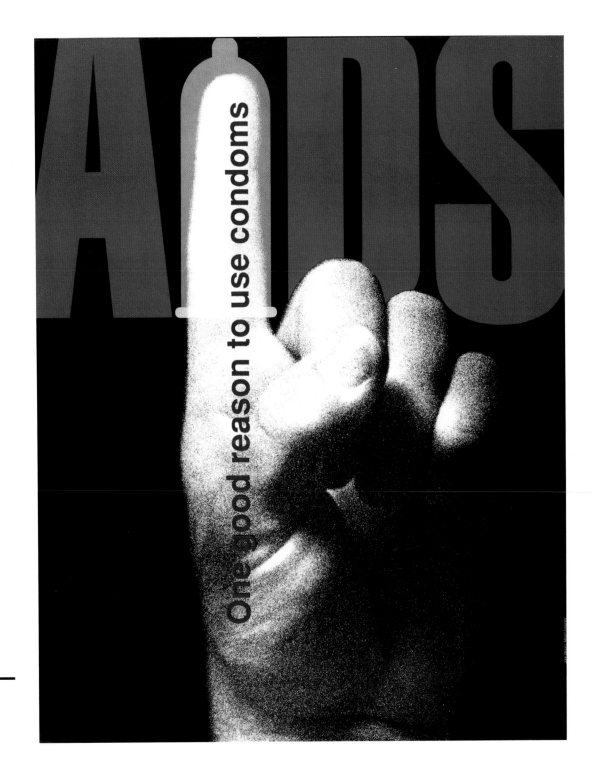

"One Good Reason to Use Condoms.
AIDS," n.d.
Alfred, New York, U.S.A.
Creator: Alfred University
Designer: John Bloom
56 x 43 cm
AP1109

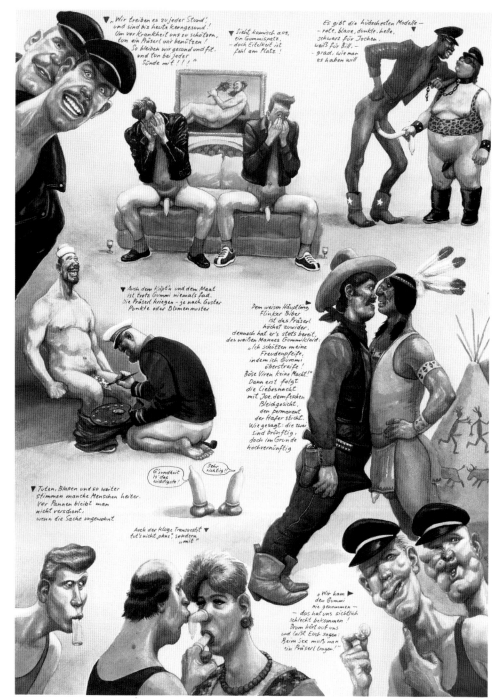

"Condoms Are the Most Important Means of Prevention" (translated from German), 1988
Vienna, Austria
Creator: AIDS-Informationszentrale Austria (AIDS-Hilfe Informationsstelle)
84 x 59 cm
AP5964

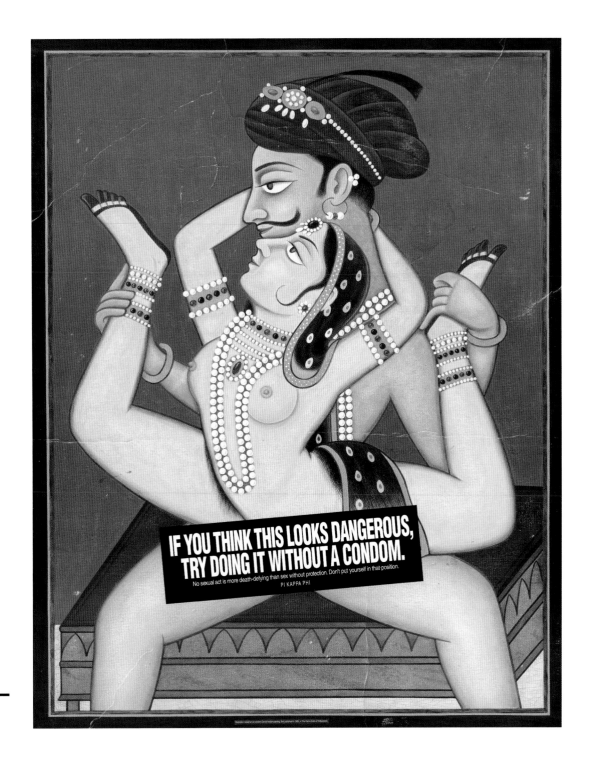

"If You Think This Looks Dangerous,
Try Doing It without a Condom," n.d.
U.S.A.
Creator: Pi Kappa Phi
73 x 57 cm
AP5176

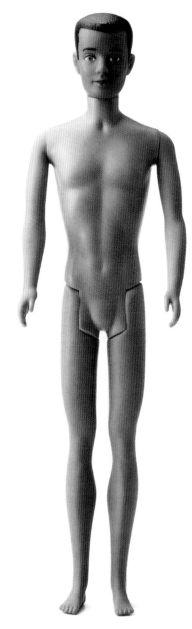

Unless You're Built Like This, You Should Be Using Condoms.

MINNESOTA AIDS PROJECT

"Unless You're Built Like This,
You Should Be Using Condoms," n.d.
Minneapolis, Minnesota, U.S.A.
Creator: Minnesota AIDS Project
Photograph: Tom Connors
65 x 43 cm
AP1793

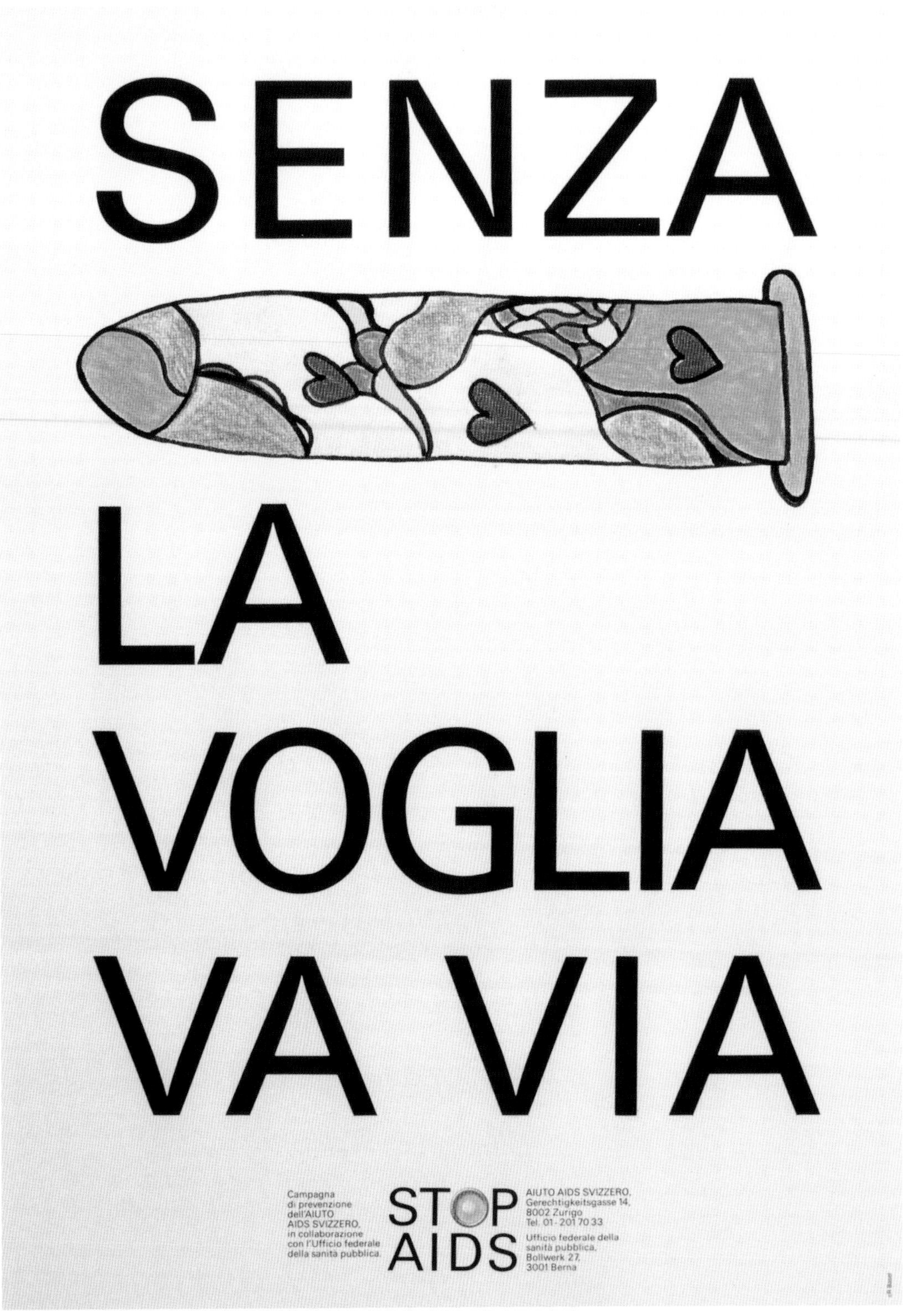

SENZA

LA VOGLIA VA VIA

"Without [a Condom] the Urge Goes Away:
Stop AIDS" (translated from Italian), 1987
Series: *Stop AIDS*
Zurich, Switzerland
Creators: AIDS-Hilfe Schweiz
Designer: Niki de Saint-Phalle
55 x 39 cm
AP5851

Campagna
di prevenzione
dell'AIUTO
AIDS SVIZZERO,
in collaborazione
con l'Ufficio federale
della sanità pubblica.

STOP AIDS

AIUTO AIDS SVIZZERO,
Gerechtigkeitsgasse 14,
8002 Zurigo
Tel. 01- 201 70 33

Ufficio federale della
sanità pubblica,
Bollwerk 27,
3001 Berna

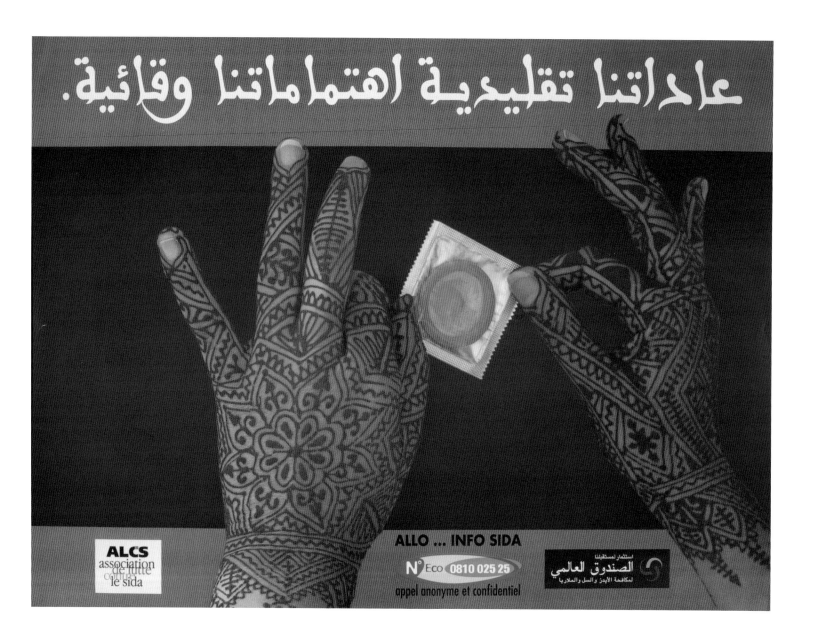

"Tradition Doesn't Rhyme with Prevention"
(translated from Arabic), 2005
Morocco
Creator: Association de lutte
contre le SIDA
48 x 64 cm
AP3597

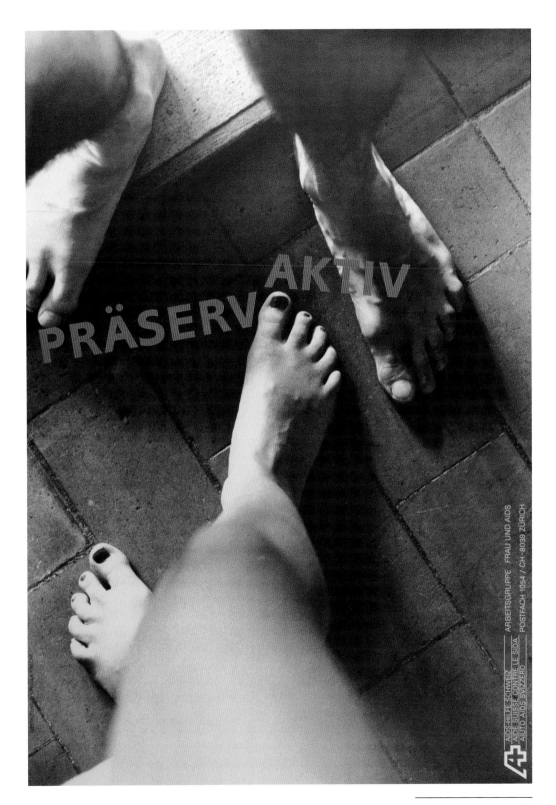

"Condom" (translated from German), 1988
Zurich, Switzerland
Creator: AIDS-Hilfe Schweiz
60 x 42 cm
AP5836

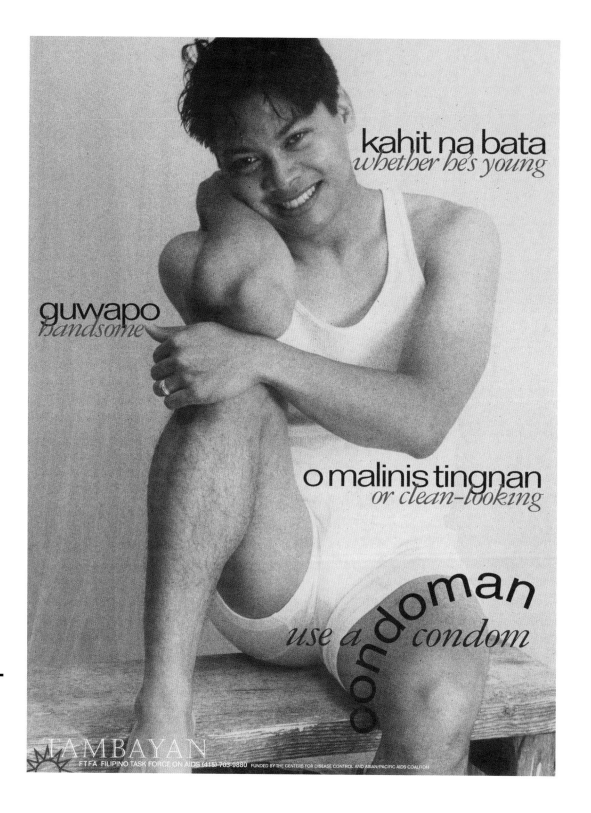

"Whether He's Young, Handsome or
Clean-Looking, Use a Condom"
(translated from Filipino), n.d.
San Francisco, California, U.S.A.
Creator: Filipino Task Force on AIDS
61 x 45 cm
AP180

Before AIDS appeared in 1981, condoms were not widely used. As Safe Sex campaigns emerged, condoms became central to the prevention discussion. Jackie Nudd, the first executive director of AIDS Rochester, the Rochester, NY AIDS community service organization, was a tireless advocate for education and safe sex. One of her earliest educational efforts was demonstrating how to put on a condom, using a banana. This image was created by a local artist for a 1983 AIDS Rochester campaign. The artist's name, unfortunately, has been lost, as has the original artwork.

The image imitates the style of Andy Warhol, the consummate pop artist of the era. Warhol's record album cover for *The Velvet Underground & Nico* (1967) was the inspiration. Even the LP vinyl disc in the original 1967 pressing was banana yellow in color.

The poster from the series *Banana Boys*, speaks to the power of art as a weapon in the AIDS war. Over the years, the image has appeared in books and magazine articles, on posters, and on the Internet as a central part of the history of the epidemic.

Copies of the poster are housed in the collections of the libraries of the National Institutes of Health, Bethesda, MD; U.S. Centers for Disease Control and Prevention; the AIDS Education Posters at the University of Rochester Department of Rare Books, Special Collections, and Preservation; and Trillium Health/AIDS Rochester archives.[1]

Dr. William M. Valenti

Dr. William M. Valenti is an infectious diseases specialist in Rochester, NY, U.S.A., and the co-founder of Community Health Network, now Trillium Health.

1. The poster is copyright AIDS Rochester/ Trillium Health, Inc., 1983. See the article, which includes the poster and the LP, at https://www.theatlantic.com/entertainment/archive/2011/12/from-haring-to-condom-man-art-as-weapon-in-the-war-against-aids/249229/ (accessed March 23, 2020).

[Banana], 1983
Series: *Banana Boys*
Rochester, New York, U.S.A.
Creator: AIDS Rochester
51 x 41 cm
AP1097

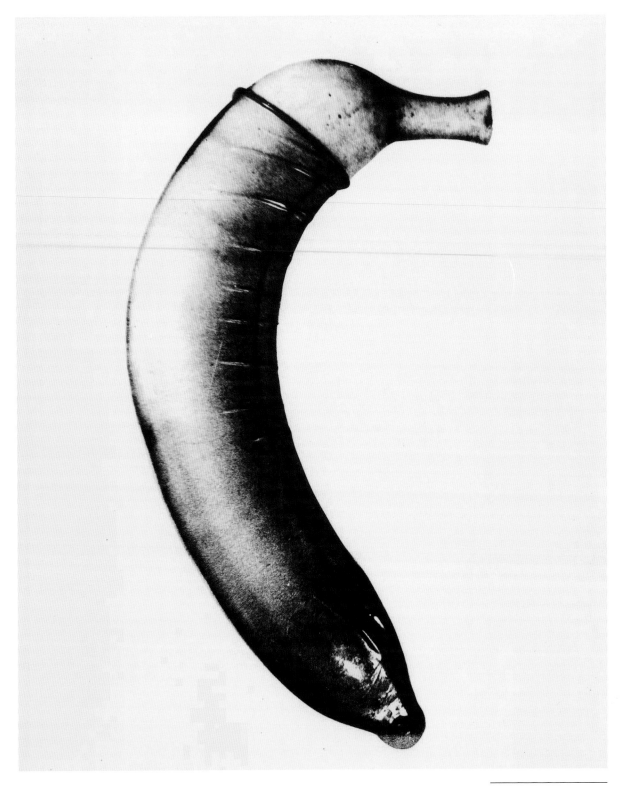

"It is time for a safer sex crusade that accepts no limits in funding or explicitness, and that refuses to accept the limits on our rights to life." [1]

The year 1992 in the UK saw a number of events that led to a resurgence of gay activism, including the "re-gaying" of HIV/AIDS and the formation of Gay Men Fighting AIDS (GMFA).

From the start, design and photography were important in establishing GMFA's credibility with its audience and positioning it as a community-based organization, producing interventions for and by gay men. Explicit imagery and language were employed not just because this would appeal to the audience, but as an intrinsic part of the activism. GMFA celebrated gay sex and deliberately rejected the visual euphemisms of mainstream AIDS health promotion.

The popular 1994 poster series featuring sailors ("Semen Kit"), a boxer ("Fight Back"), construction workers ("Build a Future"), and men in army fatigues ("Conquer AIDS") referenced fantasy gay archetypes accompanied by playful copywriting. Designed by Declan Buckley, the posters had high production values—professional quality photography by Hywel Williams,

contemporary typography[2] and full-color litho printing. GMFA was a volunteer-led grassroots organization, but these campaign materials were not photocopied amateur agitprop. Compared with some of the Health Education Authority's innocuous imagery,[3] GMFA's icons were sexualized, provocative, and pro-active representations of a gay masculinity prepared to "fight back."[4]

Siân Cook
Siân Cook is a graphic designer and senior lecturer at London College of Communication.

1. Keith Alcorn, "InSIGHT: 10,364 and counting...," *Capital Gay* (May 22, 1992).
2. The typeface used was Template Gothic, designed by Barry Deck, released by *Emigre* in 1991.
3. For example, the "Inserts" campaign, Health Education Authority, 1995. See Becky Field, Kaye Wellings, and Dominic McVey, *Promoting Safer Sex: A History of the HEA's Mass Media Campaigns on HIV, AIDS and Sexual Health 1987–1996* (London: Health Education England, 1997).
4. For some, this also challenged gay community norms: "...some men may see protected or non-penetrative sex as a threat to their masculinity. The hardline, upfront 'fighting back' campaign produced by Gay Men Fighting AIDS taps into these representations of masculinity." J.E. Stockdale and M. Dockrell, "Developing Effective Safer Sex Advertising," *The AIDS Letter,* no. 48 (April/May 1995), 2.

"Semen Kit," ca. 1994
London, England, UK
Creator: Gay Men Fighting AIDS
Designer: Declan Buckley
Photographer: Hywel Williams
59 x 42 cm
AP6182

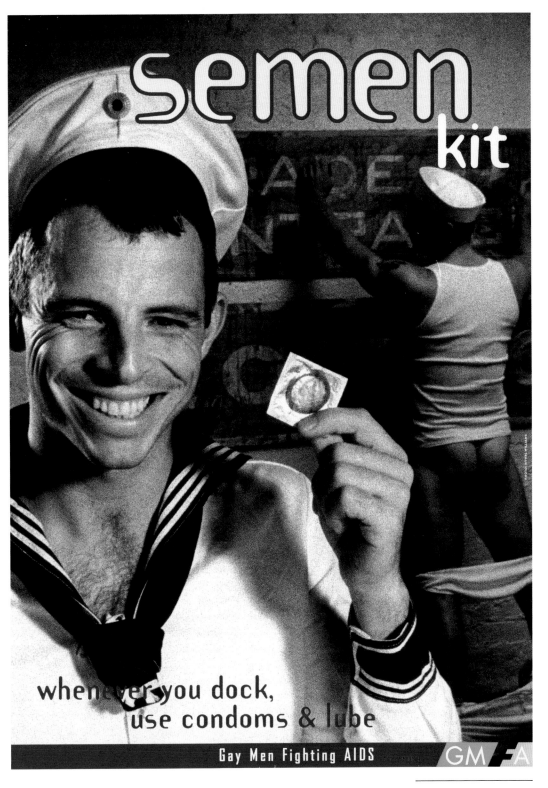

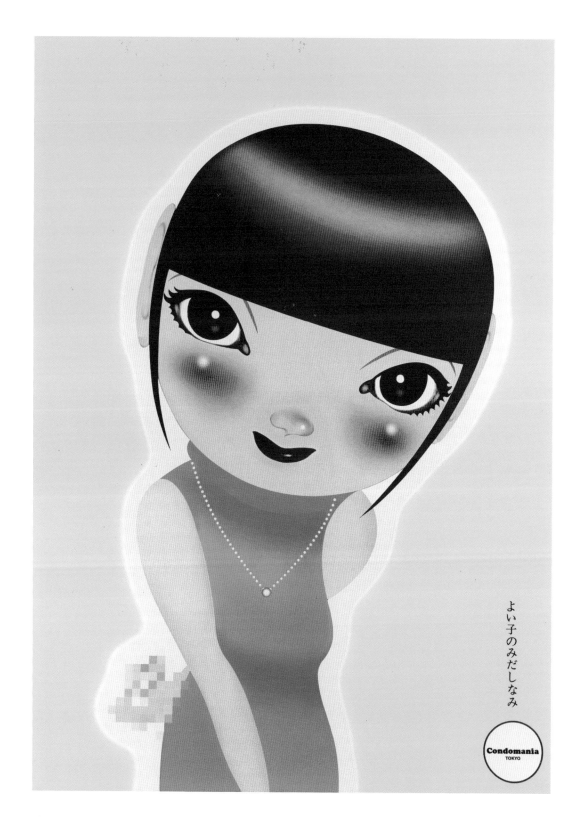

よい子のみだしなみ

Condomania
TOKYO

"Condomania: Etiquette to Prevent AIDS,"
ca. 2000
Tokyo, Japan
Designer: Akihiko Tsukamoto and
Radical Suzuki
104 x 73 cm
AP50040

158

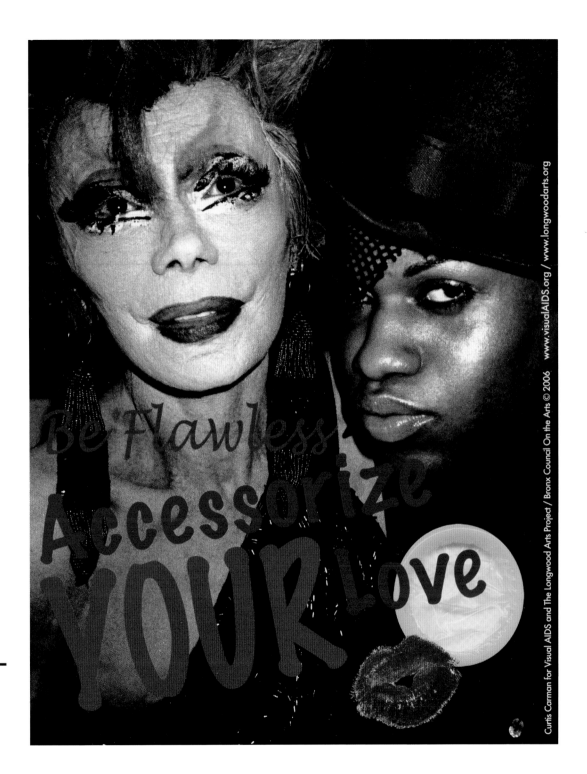

"Be Flawless. Accessorize Your Love,"
2006
Bronx, New York, U.S.A.
Creator: Visual AIDS and Bronx Council
on the Arts. Longwood Arts Project
Designer: Curtis Carmon
43 x 28 cm
AP10109_01

"AIDS. Clean Them."

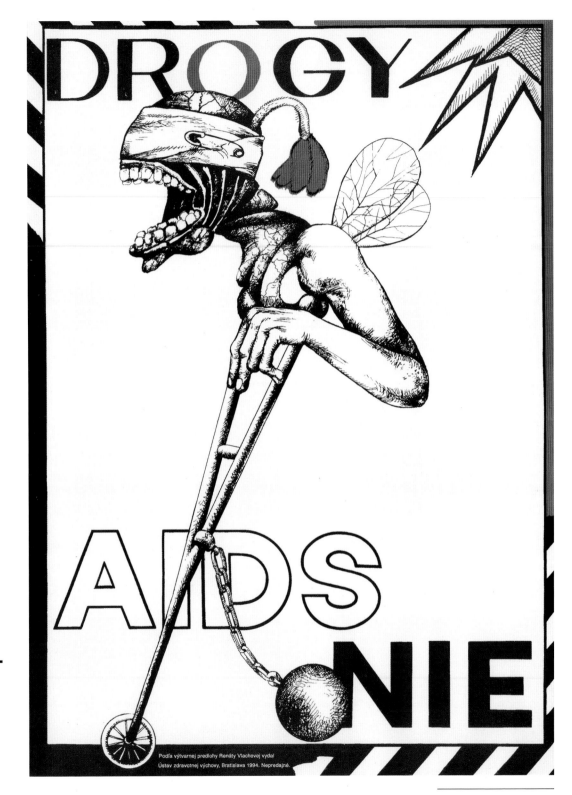

"Drugs. AIDS. Never."
(translated from Slovak), 1994
Bratislava, Slovakia
Creator: Vydal ustav zdravotnej vychovy,
Bratislava.
60 x 42 cm
AP5415

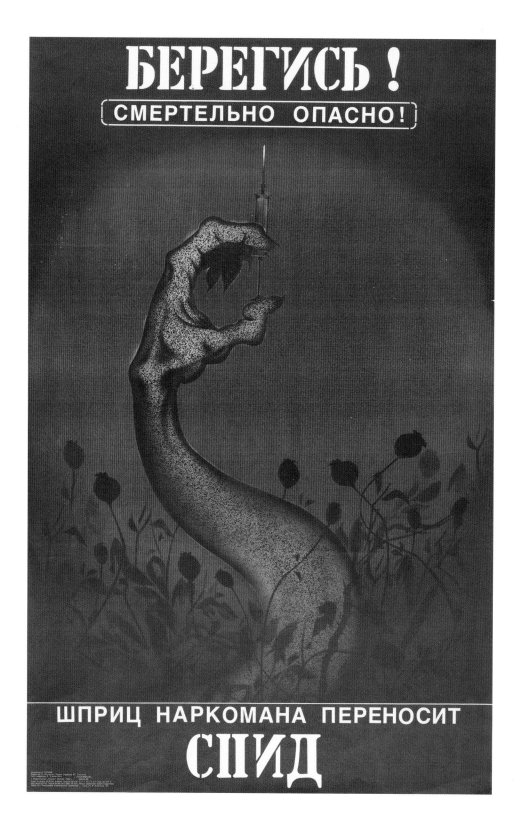

"Beware! Lethal Danger!
An Addict's Syringe Carries AIDS"
(translated from Russian), 1988
Russia
88 x 55 cm
AP5428

HOUSEHOLD HINTS FOR DRUG USERS

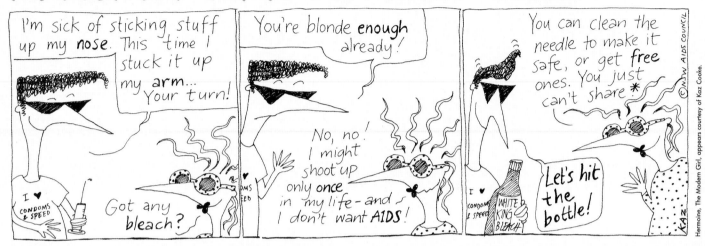

Rinse needles through TWICE with cold clean tap water, TWICE with fresh bleach, and TWICE with water again

FOR INFORMATION ABOUT NEEDLE EXCHANGES RING: **FOR INFORMATION ABOUT SAFE SEX RING:**

Produced by the AIDS Council of New South Wales with funding from the New South Wales AIDS Bureau and the Australian Federation of AIDS Organisations

"Household Hints for Drug Users," 1989
New South Wales, Australia
Creator: AIDS Council of
New South Wales
Designer: Kaz Cooke
42 x 59 cm
AP3239

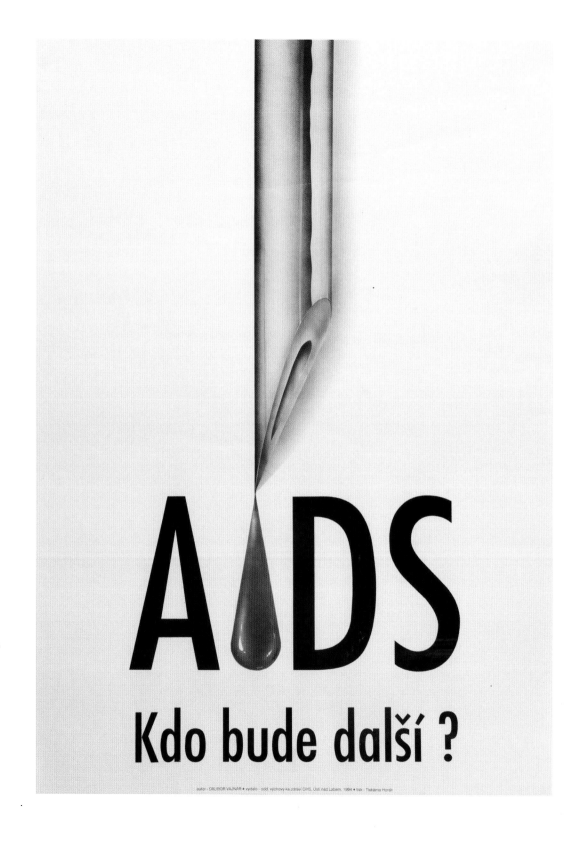

"AIDS. Who Will Be Next?"
(translated from Czech), 1994
Czech Republic
Creator: Vydalo NCPZ
(Národní centrum podpory zdraví)
(National Centre for Health Promotion)
Designer: Dalibor Vajnar
60 x 42 cm
AP5439

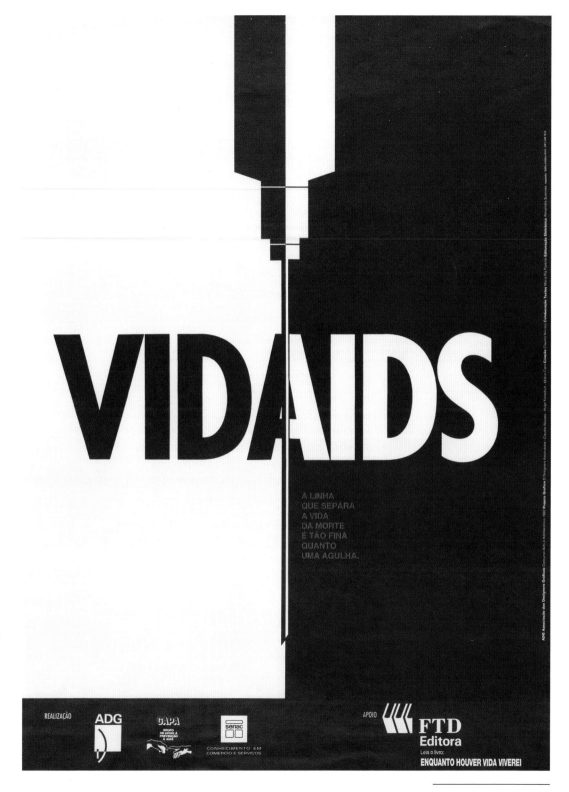

"LIFE/AIDS: The Line That Separates
Life from Death Is as Thin as a Needle"
(translated from Portuguese), 1992
Brazil
Creator: Grupo de Apoio
à Prevenção da Aids
64 x 46 cm
AP5986

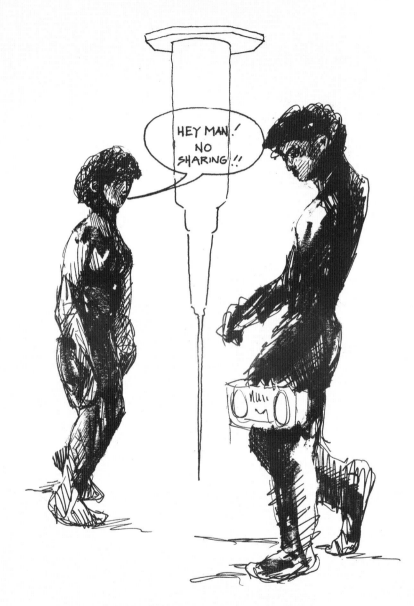

"Hey Man! No Sharing!!" n.d.
Brooklyn, New York, U.S.A.
Creator: Brooklyn AIDS Task Force
59 x 38 cm
AP1200

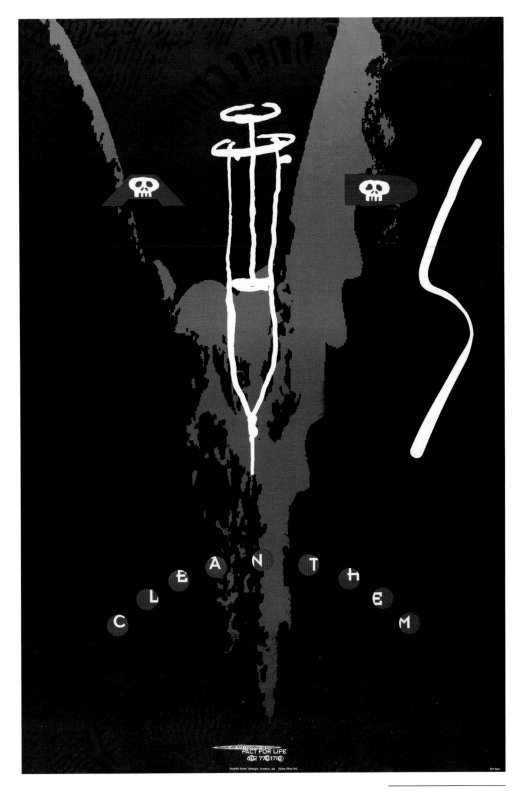

"AIDS. Clean Them," n.d.
Tucson, Arizona, U.S.A.
Creator: People with AIDS
Coalition of Tucson
97 x 64 cm
AP5207

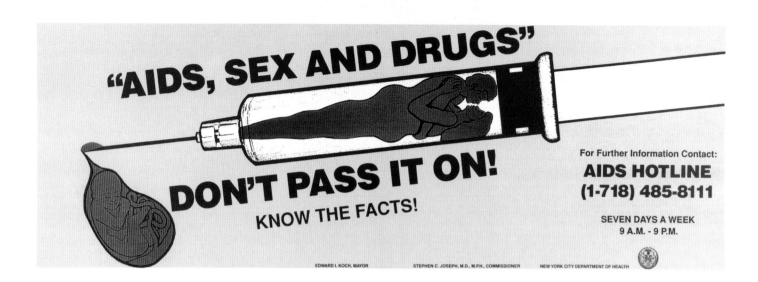

"AIDS, Sex and Drugs. Don't Pass It On!"
1987
New York, New York, U.S.A.
Creator: New York City
Department of Health
28 x 72 cm
AP1087

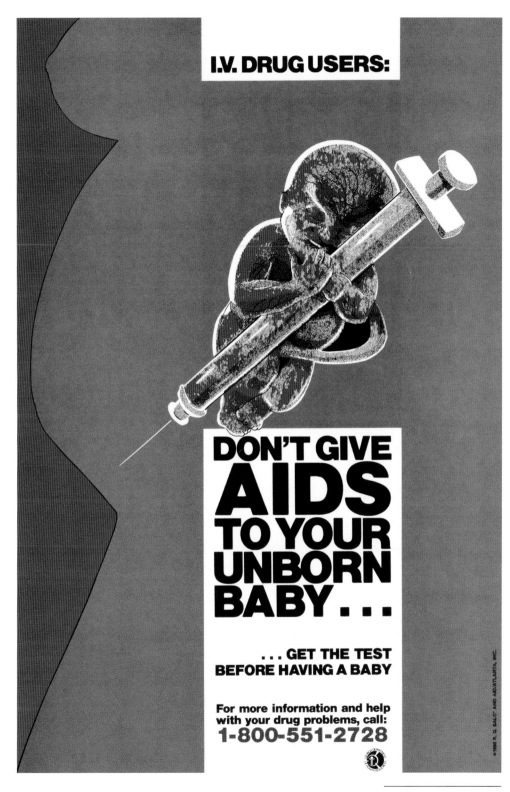

"I.V. Drug Users: Don't Give AIDS
to Your Unborn Baby," 1986
Atlanta, Georgia, U.S.A.
Creator: Georgia Department
of Human Resources
43 x 28 cm
AP2766

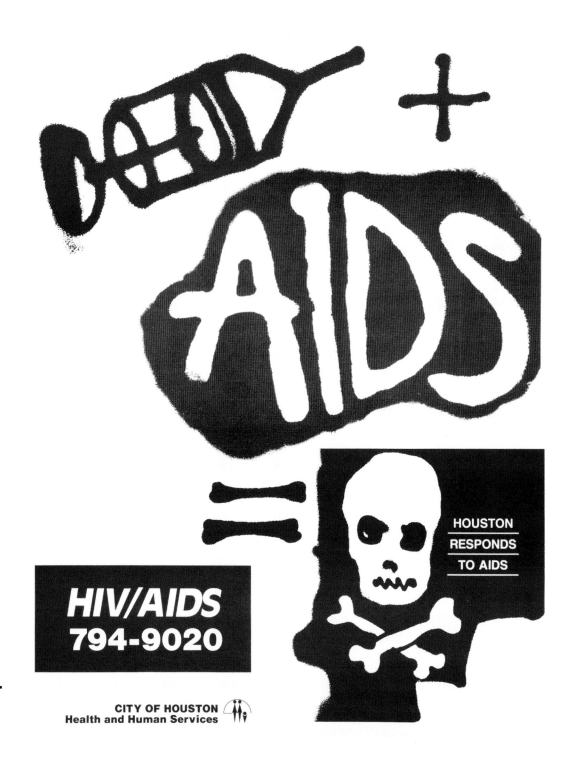

"Houston Responds to AIDS," n.d.
Houston, Texas, U.S.A.
Creator: City of Houston Health
and Human Services
56 x 43 cm
AP1707

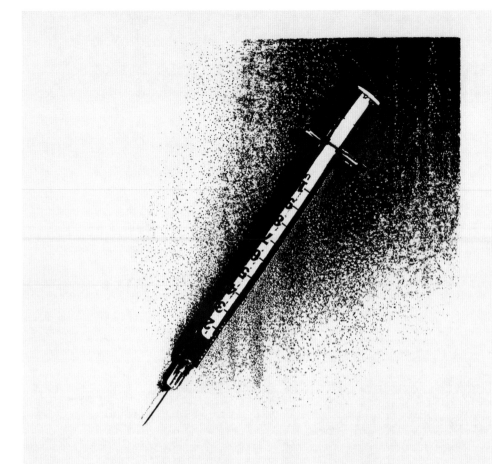

Prevent AIDS. **Exchange your needles.** Contact Prevention Point. **It could save your life.**

JUST SAY KNOW

Girl with Arms Akimbo for Prevention Point, San Francisco, 1990.

"Just Say Know," 1990
San Francisco, California, U.S.A.
Creator: Girl with Arms Akimbo,
for Prevention Point
43 x 28 cm
AP77

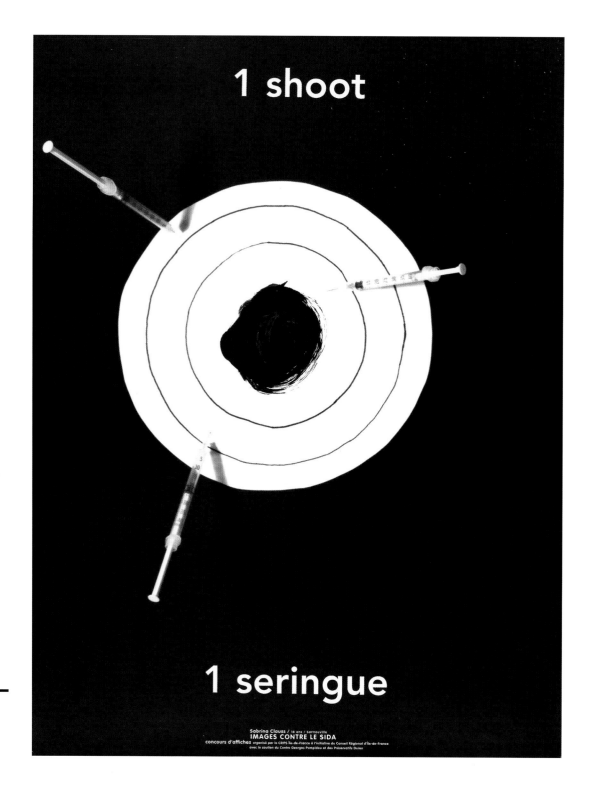

"1 Shoot, 1 Syringe"
(translated from French), n.d.
France
Creator: Images contre le SIDA
80 x 60 cm
AP6515

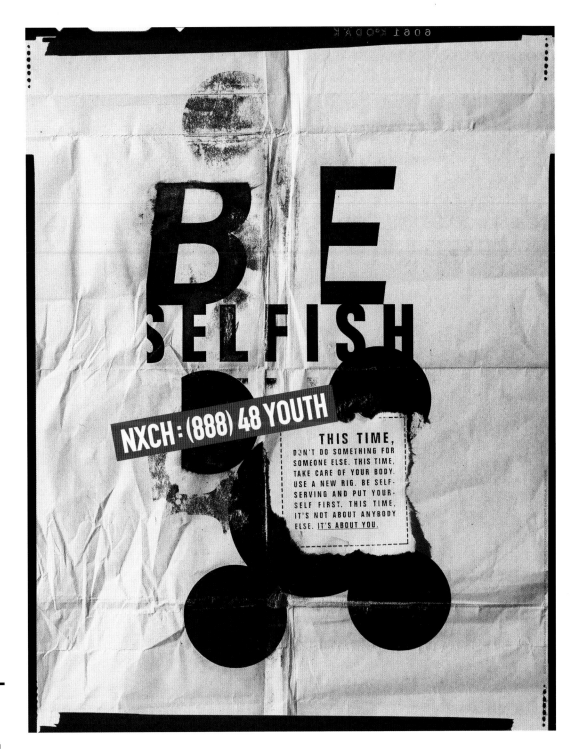

"Be Selfish," 1996
Series: *NXCH*
San Francisco, California, U.S.A.
Creator: San Francisco AIDS Foundation
59 x 45 cm
AP332

"...Blood on Its Hands."

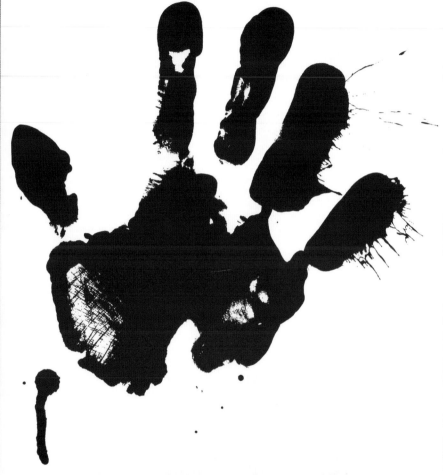

"The Government Has Blood on Its Hands.
One AIDS Death Every Half Hour," 1988
New York, New York, U.S.A.
Creator: Gran Fury
81 x 52 cm
AP1920

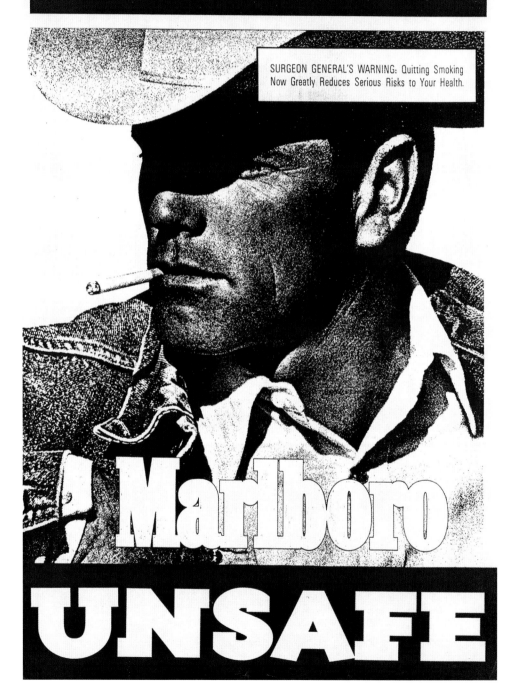

"Unsafe: Marlboro," 1990
San Francisco, California, U.S.A.
Creator: Girl with Arms Akimbo
43 x 28 cm
AP81

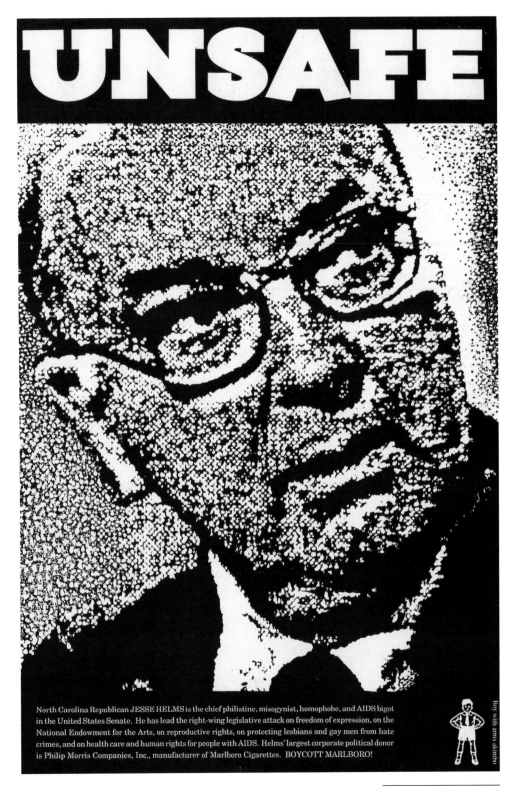

"Unsafe," 1990
San Francisco, California, U.S.A.
Creator: Boy with Arms Akimbo
43 x 38 cm
AP82

The proliferation of graphic works arising in response to the AIDS crisis marked the visual landscape with a new four-letter word that would come to define a generation "united in anger,"[1] fortified through their resistance to the very extremes of stigma, and in a love deep enough to give care to those at the very limits of life. Replacing Robert Indiana's iconic artwork *LOVE*, artists Felix Partz, Jorge Zontal, and AA Bronson, who from 1969 to 1994 comprised the Canadian collective General Idea, demanded a widespread—indeed viral—regard for AIDS in a political climate haunted by a deadly, infuriating silence. The U.S. saw AIDS made infinitely reproducible in bold text filling the volumetric void left by the refusal on the part of the Reagan administration to speak its name.

Then came AIDSGATE. Published in 1987, a scowling Reagan appears in halftone, leering from an acid yellow page, the whites of his eyes burning pink. The striking neologism is stamped across his neck in the same hot pink used for the inverted pink triangle the year before when the proclamation "Silence = Death" was made by a newly formed collective of the same name. The Silence = Death Collective went on to create the "AIDSGATE" poster, which, distributed by then-yearling ACT UP (AIDS Coalition to Unleash Power), effectively branded Reagan's violently negligent presidency. Appearing the year in which Reagan made his first major speech on AIDS, the work remains an iconic touchstone for understanding the impact of the U.S. government's silence and subsequent outright refusal to take action at the time of the crisis. Coming five years after the acronym AIDS was first acknowledged and published in the press, Reagan's first-ever speech on AIDS came with the announcement that the government would not support AIDS education efforts.[2] In the wake of this announcement, ACT UP's poster asks, "What is Reagan's *real* policy on AIDS? Genocide of all Non-whites, Non-males, and Non-heterosexuals?"

Johnny Forever Nawracaj

Johnny Forever Nawracaj is a non-binary, Polish-born multidisciplinary artist who holds an MFA from Roski School of Art and Design at the University of Southern California in Los Angeles as well as an MA in art history from Concordia University in Montréal.

1. A key phrase from ACT UP's mission statement. AIDS Coalition to Unleash Power, https://actupny. org/ (accessed July 27, 2019).
2. "Reagan's AIDSGATE," AIDS Coalition to Unleash Power, https://actupny.org/reports/reagan.html (accessed July 27, 2019.

"AIDSGATE," 1987
New York, New York, U.S.A.
Creator: Silence = Death Collective
86 x 56 cm
AP5167

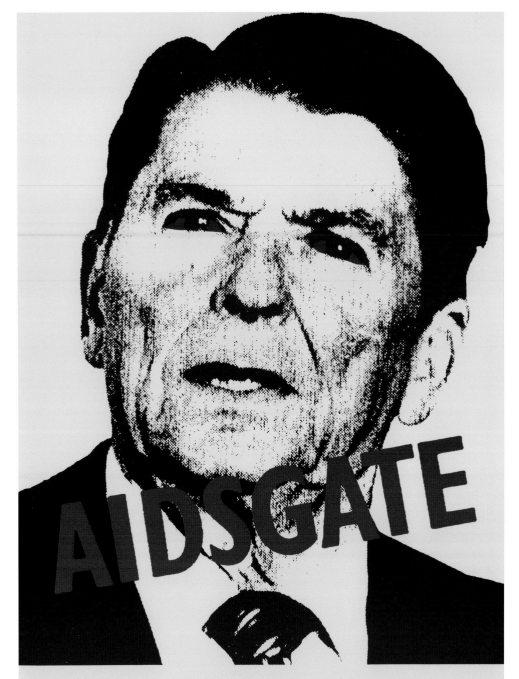

This Political Scandal Must Be Investigated!

54% of people with AIDS in NYC are Black or Hispanic... AIDS is the No. 1 killer of women between the ages of 24 and 29 in NYC... By 1991, more people will have died of AIDS than in the *entire* Vietnam War... What is Reagan's *real* policy on AIDS? Genocide of all Non-whites, Non-males, and Non-heterosexuals?...

SILENCE = DEATH

© 1987 AIDS Coalition To Unleash Power

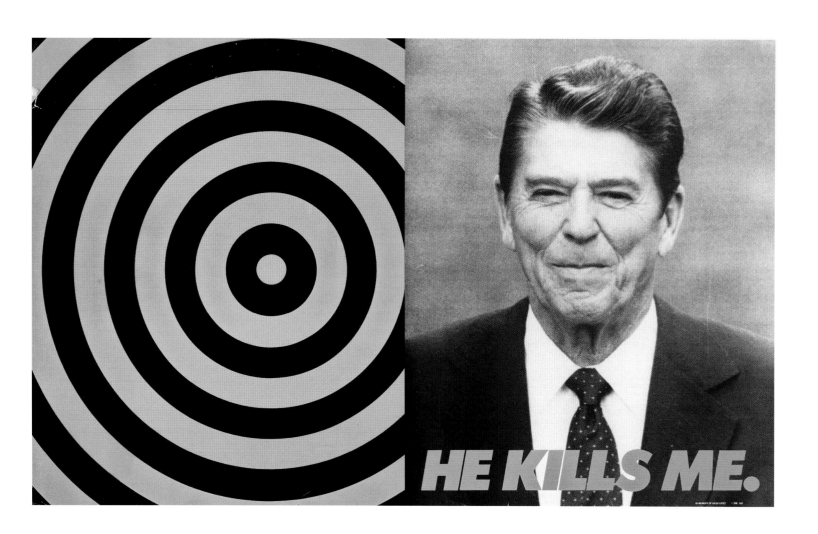

"He Kills Me," 1987
New York, New York U.S.A.
Creator: Donald Moffett
60 x 96 cm
AP8094

This was the president of the United States of America (1981–1989). For the first time ever, Ronald Reagan as pictured here appears human to me. I had friends and lovers with Kaposi lesions on their bodies and faces. I would eat with them, sleep with them, hold them in my arms, and be seen in public with them. I experienced the horror and fear that we were met with, too often then—way back when.

Some believe this is what he really looked like without makeup, evidence that he wasn't lying when he told his wife, Nancy, he'd slept with Rock Hudson to make her jealous. I read that on social media while at a conference on human sexuality. Regrettably, it wasn't true. What was true was that he chose to ignore the epidemic rather than educate the public to the health crisis. He had no concern for black or brown bodies, homosexuals, drug addicts, or the health care system that took care of them.

Despite the evidence that this was a national health crisis needing active, passionate care and funding, instead it became a reason to promote racism and homophobia. We were told we were getting what we deserved—a reason, which he disposed of with regards to his good friend Rock, who died of AIDS complications during Ronnie's term.

Too many of us were sick, our numbers growing exponentially. He showed no concern for women and even less for children, many who would seroconvert—undergo a change from a seronegative to a seropositive condition— within years after becoming sexually active. The pattern of seroconversion hasn't changed. Neither has the stigma.

Sur Rodney (Sur)

Sur Rodney (Sur) is an independent archivist, curator, and writer in New York City and Montréal.

"*Colors*," 1994
Italy
Creator: Benetton
58 x 38 cm
AP10447_01

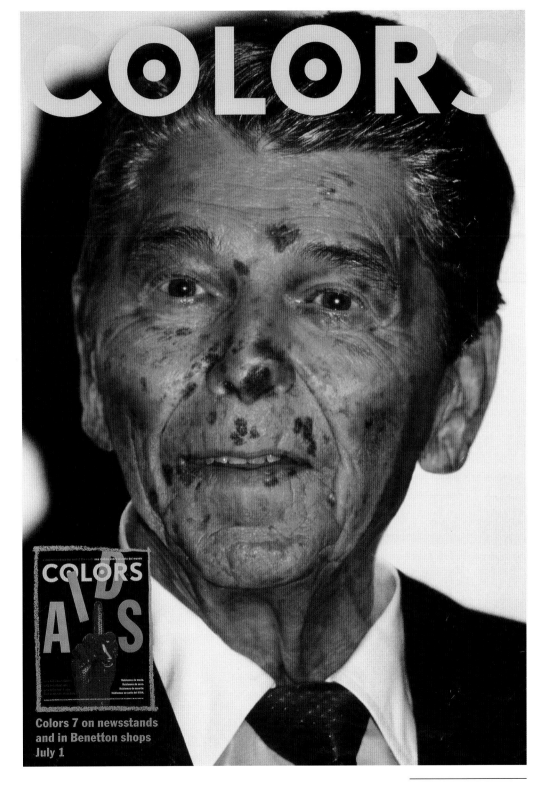

UNWANTED BY THE PEOPLE

MURDER — ARMED ROBBBERY — DRUGS
TERRORISM — COVER UP — BAD TASTE

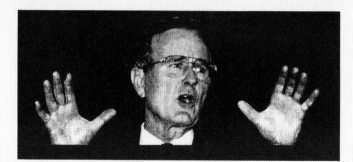

GEORGE BUSH

Name: George Herbert Walker Bush   *Age:* 66   *Eyes:* Beady Blue
Birthplaces: Milton, MA, Houston, TX, U.S.A.   *Height:* 6'2"   *Hair & Mind:* Fading
Aliases: Ronald Reagan, Manuel Noriega, Whimp   *Weight:* 205 Lbs.   *Race:* Rich White Male

MURDER — TERRORISM — DRUGS

• Bush is wanted for the murders of 9,000 Nicaraguan civilians, including 400 children. Bush was a conspirator in the Reagan Administration's dirty war against Nicaragua. The illegal airlifting of weapons to the Contra terrorists was financed in part through the sale of cocaine smuggled back into our country in the same planes. These weapons shipments were also funded by sales of arms to Ayatollah Khomeini's Iran. Meanwhile Bush served as Chairman of both the National Narcotics Border Interdiction System and the President's Task Force on Combatting Terrorism. Recently, Bush has successfully obstructed the investigation and prosecution of Iran-Contra Affair crimes, such as those of Joseph Fernandez, the ex-CIA station chief in Costa Rica.
• Bush is wanted for conspiracy in the brutal murders of six Jesuit priests by a U.S. paid hit squad in El Salvador on Nov. 16, 1989.
• He is wanted for questioning in the "under-reported" deaths and disappearances of hundreds of Panamanian civilians on or about the night of Dec. 20, 1989. He is responsible for assault on an unarmed populace with high tech terror weapons, such as Stealth bombers and laser weapons.

ARMED ROBBERY — COVER UP

• After his conversion to Reaganomics, Bush participated in the largest peacetime military buildup in U.S. history, while slashing spending on housing, education, health care, and environmental protection. He has supported the wholesale export of American industries, capital, and decent paying jobs, often to countries with repressive governments. While presiding over the decline in real wages of American workers, Bush has increased his own net worth, derived originally from offshore oil drilling, to more than two million dollars.
• With the help of the mainstream U.S. media, he has covered up the role of the CIA and the Mafia in looting now defunct Savings and Loan Institutions during the 1980's. Bush's son, Neil Bush, was a director of Silverado Springs of Denver, one of the failed S&L's linked to the CIA. Estimates of the costs to American taxpayers of the S&L bailout/ripoff are as high as 500 billion dollars.
• With the support of the Reagan Supreme Court, Bush is currently attempting to rob American women of their right to choice.

BAD TASTE

• While supporting Reagan's anti-affirmative action attacks on people of color in the U.S., Bush has applauded fascist Third World dictatorships that have trampled on human rights worldwide. In 1981 Bush told former Philippine dictator Ferdinand Marcos, "We love your adherence to democratic principles – and to the democratic process."
• Despite his claim to have "had sex" with Ronald Reagan (or was it merely "setbacks?") Bush and the Republican Party are thoroughly homophobic. They have done little to fight the AIDS epidemic or alleviate the suffering it has caused.
• While regularly referring to himself as an "environmentalist," Bush has aided and abetted big business polluters such as EXXON, hindered efforts to curb CFC and "greenhouse" gas emissions, continued potentially disastrous U.S. irrigation policies, and refused to halt the testing and development of nuclear weapons or clean up the radioactive mess this industry has created.
• Bush has repeatedly subjected the American people to public appearances by Dan Quayle.

CAUTION

• Despite his whimpish preppy demeanor, Bush is heavily armed and must be considered extremely dangerous. He served as Director of the CIA in 1976. He has known ties to the ultra right wing "secret team" of current and ex-CIA operatives who have carried out brutal campaigns against popular movements from Viet Nam to Chile. He has strong connections in the ruling sectors of corporate America.
• *Bush can be apprehended and stopped only by the organized and spirited opposition of the American people,*

"Unwanted by the People," 1990
U.S.A.
Creator: Dogs for Bush
43 x 28 cm
AP50024

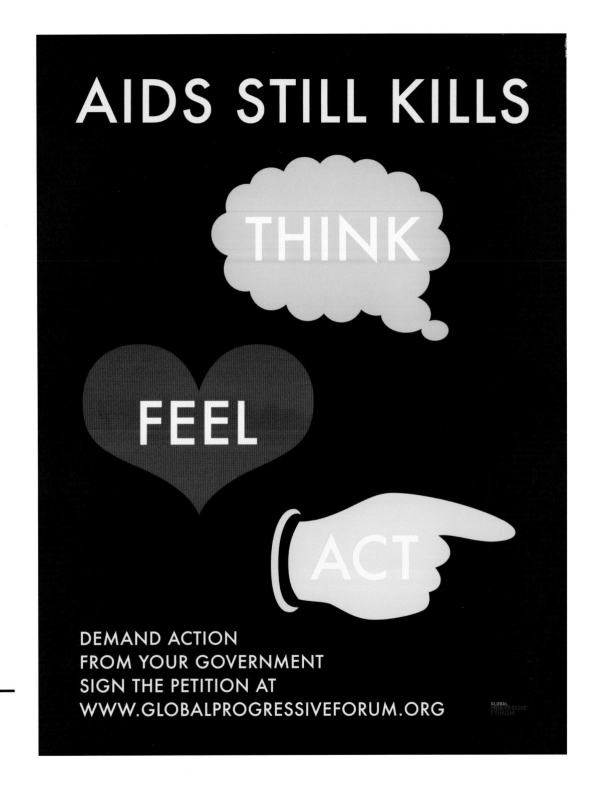

"AIDS Still Kills. Think. Feel. Act," n.d.
Brussels, Belgium
Creator: Party of European Socialists,
Global Progressive Forum
81 x 61 cm
AP11206_01

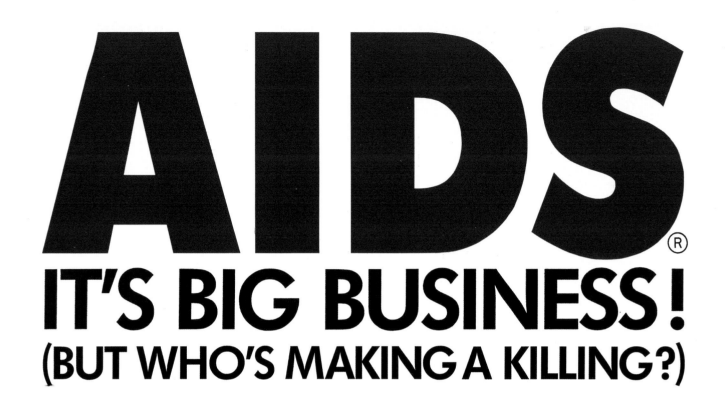

"AIDS® It's Big Business!
(But Who's Making a Killing?)," 1989
New York, New York, U.S.A.
Creator: ACT UP
28 x 57 cm
AP1330

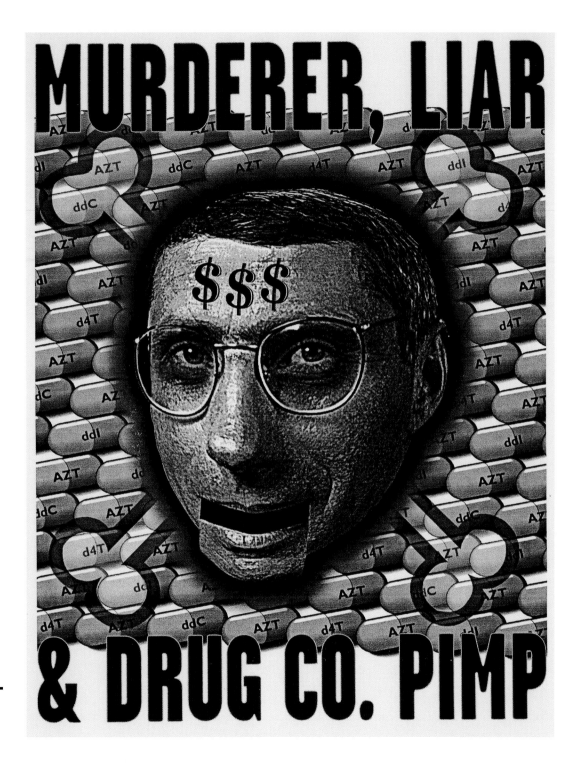

"Murderer, Liar & Drug Co. Pimp,"
  [Dr. Anthony Fauci], ca. 1996
San Francisco, California, U.S.A.
Creator: ACT UP
30 x 21.6 cm
AP13544

In 1994, Canada's Expert Committee on AIDS and Prisons released its "landmark" recommendations to address the HIV crisis in Canadian prisons. Twenty-five years later, the HIV prevalence rates in Canadian prisons are still ten times that of the general population. The problem was never a lack of ideas, it was a lack of political will. This poster by Neal Hartwick-Freeland and Giselle Dias—a collaboration across prison walls—calls us to heed the dangerous effects of that lack of political will: Prisons Kill.

For decades, the Canadian state has turned to prisons and putting people in cages as its response to a wide range of social problems—poverty, homelessness, mental health, drug use, and HIV/AIDS. In the period immediately preceding the creation of this poster, this reactionary approach was expanded. The Conservative Harper administration passed an omnibus crime bill instituting mandatory minimum sentences, slashing parole eligibility, and expanding the use of double-bunking—housing multiple prisoners in cells designed for one.

Hartwick-Freeland and Dias's poster centers the prisoner's voice amongst these issues to capture the despair, the boredom, and the anger housed within a prison system that condemns so much human potential to waste away. It holds up a mirror to the barbarism of the justice system, glimpsing an abolitionist future, and stating unequivocally the imperative for all those who dream of a better world: Kill Prisons.

Joshua Valentine Pavan

Joshua Valentine Pavan is co-founder of the Prisoner Correspondence Project, a solidarity project for queer prisoners in Canada and the United States, and outreach coordinator for the Support Staff Union at McGill University in Montréal.

"Canada's Solution to Homelessness, Drug Use, Mental Health and HIV/AIDS... Lock 'Em Up Till They Die?!" 2012
Toronto, Ontario, Canada.
Creator: AIDS Action Now!
Designers: Neal Hartwick-Freeland and Giselle Dias
30 x 46 cm
AP13595

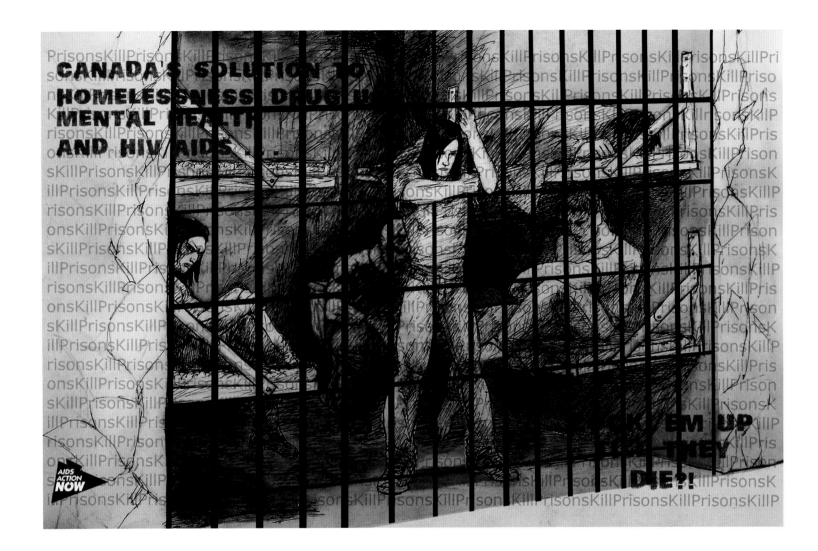

The concept for "Enjoy AZT" was originally proposed to the Gran Fury art collective during the early months of its formation in 1988, but was rejected because the collective felt uncomfortable critiquing AZT (azidothymidine), the only pharmaceutical intervention available to people living with HIV/AIDS at the time. Part of the poster's tagline, "Is This Health Care or Wealth Care?", however, was used as a subheading for one of the articles in the 1989 Gran Fury project *The New York Crimes*, and it was made into a poster for ACT UP that same year.

"Enjoy AZT" was deployed as a 13½- x 11¼-inch newsprint street poster announcing ACT UP's May 21, 1990, demonstration, Storm the N.I.H. (National Institutes of Health). At the time of its making, direct-to-consumer pharmaceutical advertising in America had yet to be deregulated and was an unfamiliar form. Squatting on an easily recognizable American commercial symbol represented a surgical visual code to explain how similar the mechanisms are for delivering a drug to the marketplace to those of other consumer products. Furthermore, the poster's text reveals a scathing rebuke of the commercial monopolies of pharmaceutical companies, a core activist critique of the drug approval process. The data in the rejoinder text were based on ACT UP fact sheets.

The poster was wheatpasted throughout Manhattan, but the longevity of this work is largely attributable to the efforts of the artist squat Bullet Space, which converted the work to a serigraph for a limited-edition fundraising portfolio for the homeless on the Lower East Side. In the context of the project *Your House Is Mine*, the "Enjoy AZT" image is an articulation of the intrinsic relationship between HIV/AIDS and gentrification, colonialization, and social displacement. The Bullet Space project captured the interest of curators and archivists, placing this version of "Enjoy AZT" into international archives and museum collections, including the Whitney Museum of American Art, The Metropolitan Museum of Art, The Museum of Modern Art, and the Victoria and Albert Museum.

Avram Finkelstein

Avram Finkelstein is a founding member of the Silence = Death and Gran Fury collectives.

I love so many things about this 1989 poster used by ACT UP (AIDS Coalition to Unleash Power)—starting with the brilliant visual literacy. The screaming loud, vitriolic rage encapsulated in the dissonant, mile-high letters "AZT." The tart inversion of "Enjoy." The didactic excoriation of the AIDS drug development process. The calling out of corporate greed.

AZT was the first AIDS drug to be approved by the FDA, in 1987 (only four years after the virus was discovered). But it was also absurdly expensive ($10,000 per year), toxic, and rapidly became ineffective due to the emergence of drug-resistant viral strains. The poster highlights the desperate need for better, more effective treatments, the impatience with excuses, and the urgency of reform.

ACT UP completely changed the playbook for patient advocacy groups. They showed the power of the visual arts in communicating ideas, and of the performing arts in gaining public/media attention.

After ACT UP stormed the National Institutes of Health in May of 1990, researchers and activists looked toward their shared goals. This resulted in greater inclusiveness and transparency on the part of scientists, and the involvement of advocates and community members in the design and implementation of clinical trials of new HIV treatments.

These changes have since been replicated in many other disease areas. They also helped to accelerate the first truly effective treatments for HIV, with the advent of a new class of AIDS drugs (the protease inhibitors) and the initiation of triple combination therapy in the mid-1990s.

But it all started with an uncompromising commitment by the medical establishment and the mobilization of public opinion using visual media such as this compelling poster.

Dr. Stephen Dewhurst

Dr. Stephen Dewhurst is an HIV/AIDS researcher and the vice dean of research at the School of Medicine and Dentistry, University of Rochester.

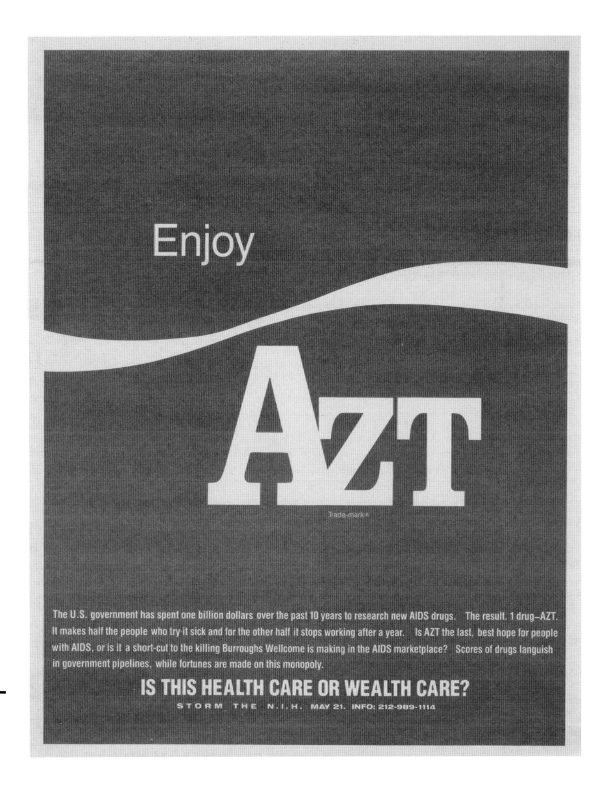

"Enjoy AZT," 1989
New York, New York, U.S.A.
Creator: Avram Finkelstein and
Vincent Gagliostro
35 x 28 cm
AP1327

Organized by the AIDS Coalition to Unleash Power (ACT UP New York) and Women's Health Action and Mobilization (WHAM!), the Stop the Church protest targeted Cardinal John O'Connor, head of the Roman Catholic Church in New York City, for his disparaging remarks about homosexuality, his opposition to comprehensive sex education in public schools, his refusal to allow church-run health care facilities to provide safer sex education and condoms, and his encouragement of anti-abortion activism. The Roman Catholic Church received public funds to run its health care facilities, which included, to activists' consternation, the first comprehensive AIDS ward in New York City.

On December 10, 1989, 4,500 protestors massed outside the landmark St. Patrick's Cathedral on Fifth Avenue, while several hundred entered the cathedral and disrupted the mass, staging a "die-in" in the aisles and shouting at Cardinal O'Connor. This was the largest and most controversial of ACT UP New York's protests, but the uses of civil disobedience and spectacular street theater were hallmarks featured in many other ACT UP demonstrations.

ACT UP members wheatpasted hundreds of copies of posters, including this one, across New York City to publicize demonstrations like Stop the Church but also to challenge homophobic framings of the AIDS epidemic. The posters also helped recruit members to the group, which offered a supportive community to those ravaged by both the AIDS epidemic and the social stigma surrounding it.

Tamar W.Carroll

Tamar W. Carroll, Ph.D., is associate professor and chair, Department of History, Rochester Institute of Technology.

"Stop the Church," 1989
Series: *Stop the Church*
New York, New York, U.S.A.
Creator: ACT UP
Designer: Vincent Gagliostro
43 x 28 cm
AP1326

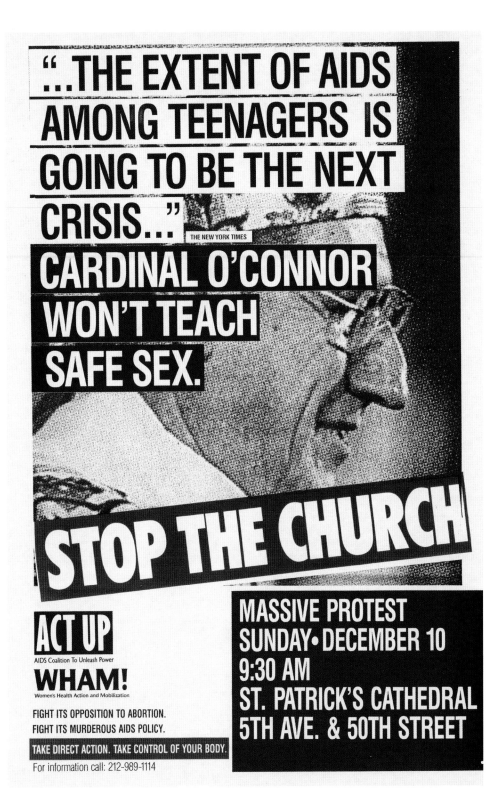

"...THE EXTENT OF AIDS AMONG TEENAGERS IS GOING TO BE THE NEXT CRISIS..." THE NEW YORK TIMES

CARDINAL O'CONNOR WON'T TEACH SAFE SEX.

STOP THE CHURCH

ACT UP
AIDS Coalition To Unleash Power

WHAM!
Women's Health Action and Mobilization

FIGHT ITS OPPOSITION TO ABORTION.
FIGHT ITS MURDEROUS AIDS POLICY.

TAKE DIRECT ACTION. TAKE CONTROL OF YOUR BODY.

For information call: 212-989-1114

MASSIVE PROTEST
SUNDAY•DECEMBER 10
9:30 AM
ST. PATRICK'S CATHEDRAL
5TH AVE. & 50TH STREET

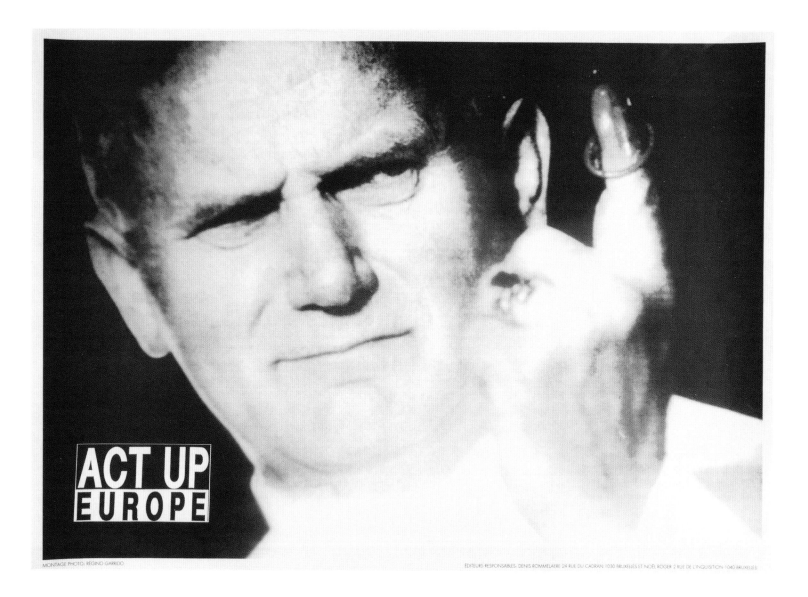

MONTAGE PHOTO: RÉGINO GARRIDO

EDITEURS RESPONSABLES: DENIS ROMMELAERE 24 RUE DU CADRAN 1030 BRUXELLES ET NOËL ROGER 2 RUE DE L'INQUISITION 1040 BRUXELLES

"ACT UP Europe," [Pope John Paul II],
ca. 1993
Paris, France
Creator: ACT UP Paris
Designers: Denis Rommelaere
and Noël Roger
44 x 61 cm
AP6571

"Action = Life"
(translated from Portuguese), 1996
Rio de Janeiro, Brazil
Creator: Grupo pela Vidda
63 x 42 cm
AP4144

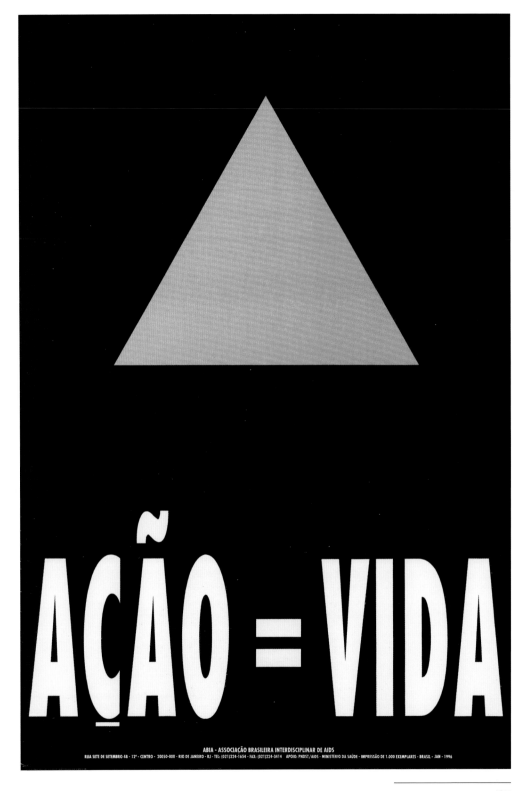

This poster was conceptualized for AIDS Action Now! in 2013, and it continues to demand an honest appraisal of progress in the lives of people living with HIV and AIDS. Initially this poster was designed to critique romantic and de-politicized notions of the history of AIDS. The poster went on to have a life of its own, inspiring confrontations and conversations between generations of activists. Younger activists, like Vincent Chevalier and me, seemed to intuitively understand the inherent dangers of a progressive narrative of AIDS history given our own continuing experience with the primarily biomedical response to what has always been a social problem. At the same time, an older generation of activists saw the poster as an assault on losses only they could truly understand—of friends, lovers, family, and the whole generation of people who died of AIDS and took with them the gifts they could have offered to the future.

This poster continues to demand two fundamental questions: who is responsible for producing, critiquing, and passing on this history? And, what is the value of the epidemic's history to its present and future? Confrontations and conversations must answer both. Ultimately, like all history, the story of AIDS must be woven from the diversity of voices who lived through it. From that dynamic interaction of voices, a sense of where the epidemic has taken us emerges and that confrontation should map our way to the future.

Ian Bradley-Perrin

Ian Bradley-Perrin is a Ph.D. candidate in Sociomedical Sciences at Columbia University Mailman School of Public Health in New York City.

"Your Nostalgia Is Killing Me!" 2013
Montréal, Québec, Canada
Creator: PosterVirus and
AIDS Action Now!
Designers: Ian Bradley-Perrin
and Vincent Chevalier
28 x 43 cm
AP 50077

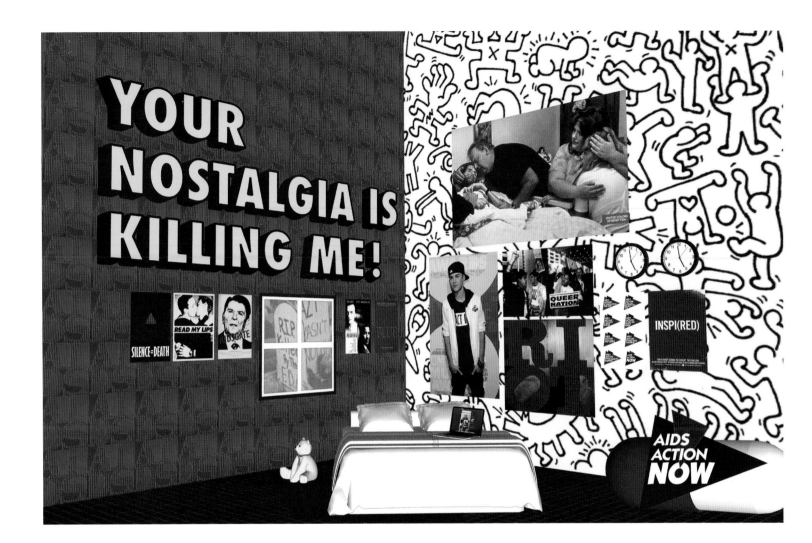

Before the HIV/AIDS pandemic, it was neither typical nor acceptable for anyone to question the medical decisions made by physicians and scientists. The AIDS activists forced that change. They felt the urgency of the AIDS crisis and used unconventional, confrontational tactics to make their voices heard. As a result, patient and constituency advocacy gained an unprecedented level of impact, as it should have.

The interactions I had with ACT UP and others in the activist community during the AIDS crisis were transformational. In those early years at the National Institutes of Health, activists in costumes held several provocative demonstrations, blowing whistles and throwing smoke bombs. During one protest, I looked at the demonstrators on the lawn from my office window above, and I sensed they were truly hurting; they were in pain and terrified. I realized that if I were in their shoes, I would do anything to be heard, just as they were doing. So against the advice of my colleagues, I brought their leaders up to talk about their concerns.

The activists had always been pushed away because of their confrontational tactics. However, by looking past the theatrics and listening carefully to what they had to say, I quickly saw that their concerns were valid, and their ideas had considerable merit. They wanted a voice in the decisions regarding the conduct of research, better access to drugs, and more flexibility in the clinical trial and regulatory processes. From that first conversation, over time, we made major changes in the way that we designed clinical trials according to the needs of the patients as well as considerably shortening the approval time for lifesaving drugs for those in dire need of treatment.

Dr. Anthony S. Fauci

Dr. Anthony S. Fauci is an immunologist and director of the National Institute of Allergy and Infectious Diseases.

"Silence = Death," 1986
New York, New York, U.S.A.
Creator: Silence = Death Collective
86 x 56 cm
AP1932

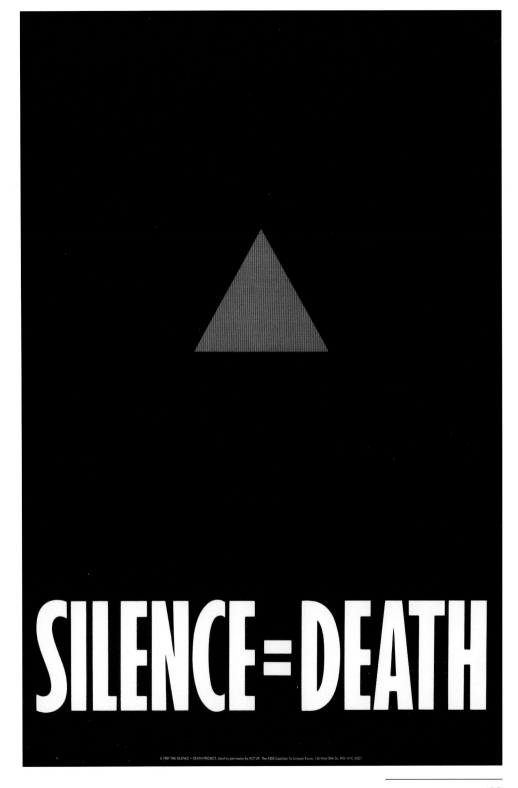

© 1987 THE SILENCE = DEATH PROJECT. Used by permission by ACT UP, The AIDS Coalition To Unleash Power, 135 West 29th St., #10, NYC 10001

"The criminalization of HIV-positive people perpetuates stigma and prevents HIV prevention. HIV-positive people are often caught in a "Catch 22," wherein disclosure is required by law but often leads to immediate rejection. Inform yourself: overcome stigma and get laid!"

That's the fine print of my 2012 poster produced by AIDS Action Now!, and it is probably the most overlooked aspect of this piece of agit-prop. I pitched the idea to PosterVirus creators Alexander McClelland and Jessica Whitbread as a way to expand on my April 2012 poem "The New Equation," which reimagines the iconic Silence = Death meme in the context of HIV disclosure and criminalization at the dawn of the U = Utopian era. Looking back on my poster and its frequent misinterpretations, I am prompted to consider how it also fits into a history of the use of "fine print" in the AIDS poster repertoire.

Like "Silence = Death," "AIDS Is Over, Right?" employs the uncanniness of a bold sentence to incite the viewer to consider who is speaking, and why, and hence to read the more didactic text below. The impact intended by the Silence = Death Collective's 1986 poster was clearly for it to function as a *détournement* of the visual language of advertising. Its use of the pink triangle, white lettering, and morbid black background

has been extensively written about, and its iconic status was so recognizable that by 2012 I thought it was finally ripe for a remake. Granted, countless remakes had already been proposed the world over—e.g., in the same year, a graffitied stencil appeared in Vancouver, Canada, that read "Silence = Breath" perhaps as an ad for a yoga studio—but none of them had spoken of my experience as an HIV-positive person.

The Visual AIDS event series *Day without Art,* celebrated on World AIDS Day since 1989, significantly chose to play with the fine print for its tenth anniversary poster, titled "AIDS Is Over, Right?" The fine print of this minimalist text-and-logo oversize poster contains a barrage of facts and stats interspersed with the red-lettered phrase "Ignorance is bliss." In a classic emotional twist, of course, nothing is "blissful" about any of these statistics, especially insofar as increased public misinformation and HIV transmission rates are concerned. What have we here other than a critical and effective use of that notorious New York weapon: sarcasm?

"Silence = Sex" picks up where "AIDS Is Over, Right?" left off. My twenty-first-century viewers, whether in Toronto, Montréal, Berlin, San Francisco, or Paris, where the poster was eventually shown in various exhibitions, were aware of the original I was riffing on, but may not

have been aware that Canadian law continued to criminalize non-disclosure. Furthermore, my point was that the very fact of criminalization is why many HIV-positive people did not want to disclose to all of their sex partners. The challenge of "or maybe you should read the fine print" underlies my poster and its two precedents, but with different levels of uncanniness. Without the fine print, we might have to reprint them as "Ignorance = Death," "AIDS Is Not Over, Please See Below," and "Sorry I Didn't Disclose That Time: Blame Canadian Jurisprudence."

Jordan Arseneault

Jordan Arseneault is an artist, translator, and co-founder of the activist collective SéroSyndicat in Montréal.

"Silence = Sex," 2012
Montréal, Québec, Canada
Creator: PosterVirus and
AIDS Action Now!
Designer: Jordan Arseneault
43 x 28 cm
AP 50076

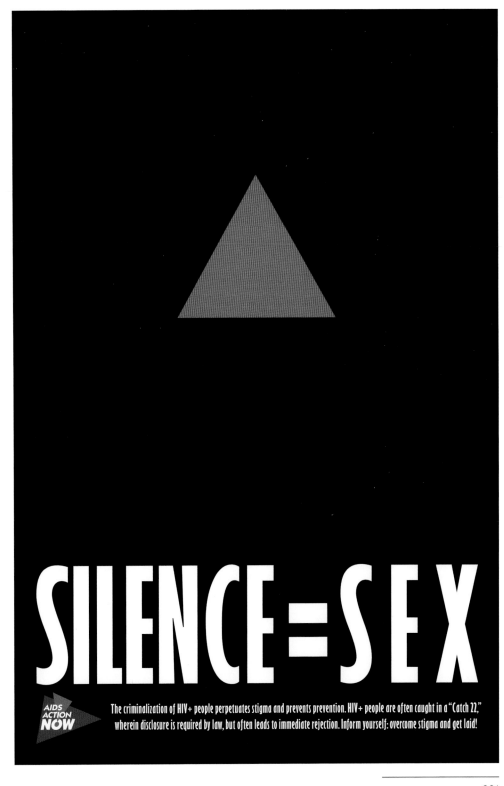

SILENCE=SEX

AIDS
ACTION
NOW

The criminalization of HIV+ people perpetuates stigma and prevents prevention. HIV+ people are often caught in a "Catch 22," wherein disclosure is required by law, but often leads to immediate rejection. Inform yourself: overcome stigma and get laid!

The Collection

Jessica Lacher-Feldman

"I saw an orange poster that showed two disem-bodied hands opening a condom wrapper when I was riding the red line, the one that runs from true Boston to Harvard. I thought that was remarkable. It was about 1990, and, when I was in medical school 35 years earlier, it was illegal to teach anything about contraception. The one lecture we had, I recall vividly, they made a lot of hoop-de-doo. We closed the doors and acted as if the police were about to raid the place. In those days, that was illegal and forbidden, and so I thought that poster was really striking. I went home, called the public health department, and said, 'Could you send me some of these posters?' And they did. That's how I started."[1]*

—Dr. Edward C. Atwater

In the superhero world, Dr. Edward Atwater's experience in that Boston subway car during the first decade of the AIDS crisis would be called his "origin story"—the beginning of a nearly thirty year quest in which he amassed the largest collection of AIDS education post-ers in the world. In the years after he saw that first poster, it is easy to imagine him boarding airplanes with his beloved wife, Ruth, wrangling cardboard tubes filled with posters up the aisle with a good-natured and earnest smile, and perhaps wearing a bowtie and sweater. While it is certain that the Atwaters' foreign travels included concert halls, fine restaurants, theaters, and museums, any trip, no matter where, most certainly also involved health clinics, community centers, and other places of advocacy and treatment in search of AIDS posters to add to the collection. And for the posters he didn't cart back from trips himself, or corresponded with organizations directly to obtain them, he dep-utized neighbors, friends, colleagues, and their children to help out.

It was in 2007 that Dr. Atwater began to give this important collection to the University of Rochester. The University was his undergrad-uate alma mater, as well as his place of employ-ment for decades as a doctor and professor of medicine. The collection was added to the River Campus Libraries' Department of Rare Books, Special Collections, and Preservation. This gift to the University of Rochester is a staggeringly significant collection. It includes posters and related ephemera aimed towards educating people from all walks of life about HIV/AIDS prevention, risks, social advocacy, and compas-sion for those affected, both the individuals who suffer and those who love them. And while Dr. Atwater did not want this important collection to bear his name, it is critical that we recognize and pay homage to his vision and foresight in build-ing the collection, beginning at that *a-ha moment* on the subway.

The AIDS Education Posters collection is astounding in its diversity and scope. It consists of more than 8,000 posters from 130 countries, in 76 languages and counting. In addition to the posters, the collection is made up of a sig-nificant array of HIV/AIDS-related ephemera, including branded condoms, fliers, booklets, postcards, and items of clothing, such as nov-elty socks with condom pockets. As a driven collector, Dr. Atwater included meticulous documentation and correspondence that shed light on how he tirelessly sought HIV/AIDS materials from across the globe. It is clear from the collection, and from knowing him and how he worked, that he didn't want to just collect some AIDS posters; he was focused and driven to create the most significant collection of its kind, because he saw a need to document this global crisis for posterity.

At the time of his gift of posters, Dr. Atwater had already been a donor and collaborator with the Miner Library Special Collections, which is part of the University of Rochester's Medical School. He gave them a substantive collection of material relating to popular medicine. Dr. Atwater was a born collector, and anecdotes relayed by him and by those who knew him leave no doubt to that assertion. Archivists and special collections librarians so value the people like Dr. Atwater in this world. His efforts, with passion and dedication, are something not easily duplicated in the archives. Moving for-ward, we will continue to build and acquire AIDS education posters , but without the personal vision that served as the genesis for the col-lection. The vision of Dr. Atwater remains and is instilled in the corpus of the materials, as well as in the way those who had the opportunity to learn from him.

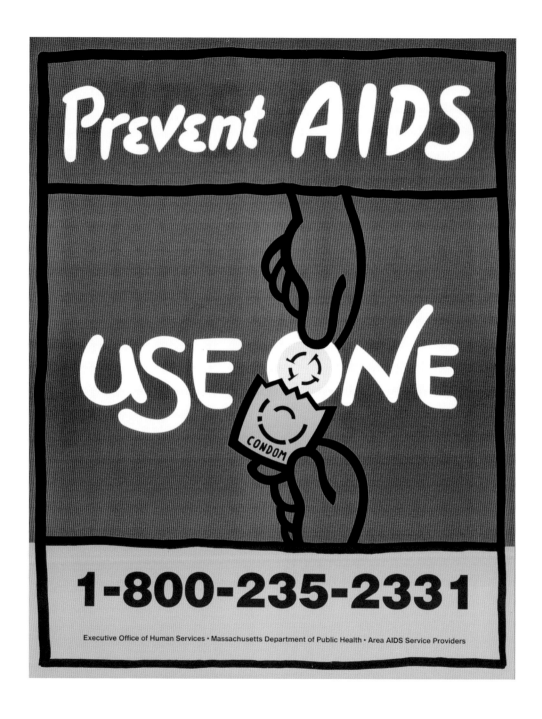

"Prevent AIDS. Use One," ca. 1991
Boston, Massachusetts
Creator: Massachusetts Department
of Public Health
56 x 43.5 cm
AP791

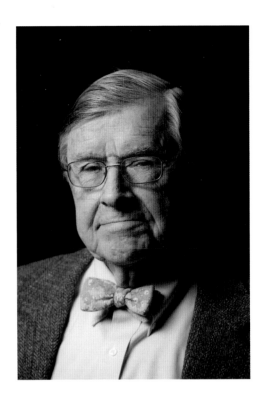

Dr. Edward C. Atwater
Photo by J. Adam Fenster,
University of Rochester

"Stop AIDS," ca. 2000
China
Designer: Shaohua Chen
86 x 60 cm
AP 50078

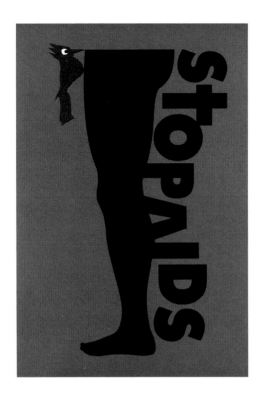

The AIDS Education Posters collection began with that chance observation around 1990, when Dr. Atwater was sixty-four years old, and he continued collecting voraciously, with perseverance and passion, until the very end of his life. In the spring of 2019, just a few weeks before his passing at the age of ninety-three, he added to the collection after a trip to New York City. This visit was punctuated by visits to Lincoln Center and The Metropolitan Museum of Art, as well as to an upscale gallery specializing in posters, where he procured a few important historic posters for the collection. His enthusiasm for building the collection was evident in acquiring a poster from Iran and one from China.

It was Dr. Atwater's personal triumph to document through these posters how messages about HIV/AIDS have been disseminated to different audiences and populations around the world from the very beginnings of the pandemic through today. Dr. Atwater was fascinated by how sensitive topics such as intimacy, sexually transmitted disease, contraception, homosexuality, sex work, pre-marital sex, and aggressive political and social protest were conveyed in these posters. They all speak to much more than the AIDS crisis, they speak to dramatic shifts in our cultural and social history at the end of the twentieth century.

My visits with Dr. Atwater were always energetic and lively. They were full of conversations on a wide range of topics—the posters, of course, as well as library projects, university politics, history, theater, classical music, dinner plans, and recent visits to the movies. My last visit to his home was punctuated by a walk to the car, boxes in tow, accompanied by Dr. Atwater using a cane, but still spry and graceful. The spring weather was coming, and he talked of the horse chestnut tree hanging over his driveway, and how against the better judgment of others, he had nursed it back to health, rather than cut it down. While looking at the tree, he cocked his head and narrowed his eyes, spotting a woodpecker in one of the upper branches. Life and art collided; one of my boxes held a rare Chinese poster that he had bought on his last trip to New York City and that included an image of a stylized woodpecker. This quiet experience was one that reminds us to take time to nurture inquiry, to observe the world around us, and to be open to what comes our way. This encounter summed up my very important three-year relationship with a donor who had become a friend.

Working in special collections librarianship exposes one to all types of people and all types of materials. When working with donors, one grows to understand an important element that is not always appreciated outside of the archival realm: when donors give materials to archives and special collections, they often have a very significant and complex attachment to these donations. Archivists work with donors who are turning over the custody of personal or family papers, or business records relating to the work of an individual. That connection, which is a post-custodial relationship with materials, does not mean that the person who once had them didn't care about them; they are just moving their materials to a different state, a different function, where they can be used, enjoyed, studied, and appreciated by a wider audience. These materials are saved, but not necessarily "collected" by the donor. A deep passion often resides in materials that were part of a family history generated during the course of lifetimes—materials such as scrapbooks, photo albums, letters, and diaries.

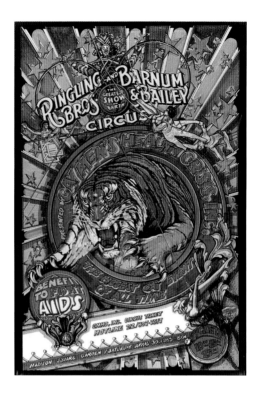

"Ringling Bros. and Barnum & Bailey
Circus: A Benefit to Fight AIDS," 1983
New York, New York, U.S.A.
Creator: Gay Men's Health Crisis
Designer: Enno Poersch
88 x 58 cm
AP50005

Dr. Edward C. Atwater
Photo by J. Adam Fenster,
University of Rochester

A rheumatologist by training, Edward Atwater was not an immunologist or a specialist in communicable diseases. But his interest in the history of medicine and how medical information is presented to the public, as well as his ability to recognize the significance of the HIV/AIDS crisis early on is what allowed him to begin to build this collection. He saw these posters as a mechanism for exploring social history even more so than medicine. An example is one of the earliest posters in the collection, which was acquired only in 2018. This poster publicized a fundraiser for the Gay Men's Health Crisis to be held at the Ringling Brothers and Barnum and Bailey Circus in New York City. The event, dated May 1983, was a "Benefit to Fight AIDS" and touted as "The Biggest Gay Event of All Time." The poster itself belied the fear and tension that gripped the city at the time, as well as other large metropolitan areas with significant communities of gay men, where something that was first known as "gay cancer" was occurring in the community. Left unchecked, the virus was causing rampant, rapid, tragic, and painful death. This poster, from the very beginning of the AIDS crisis as we know it, did little to predict what was to come in terms of the myriad messages and images that would be developed around the world to bring the disease, and ways to prevent it, to the global audience.

The collection has been a catalyst for research, and has driven numerous projects by University of Rochester graduate and undergraduate students. It has inspired exhibitions and public programming. As one of the conditions of Dr. Atwater's gift, the collection has also been made fully available online. A significant investment from the University of Rochester's River Campus Libraries has meant that the posters can be seen, used, downloaded, and shared by anyone with Internet access and a computer or device to view them. This assertion by Dr. Atwater speaks to his continuous passion about the collection and its use. It was putting the posters in a searchable online interface and creating robust metadata around the collection that allowed users to compare and contrast messages and imagery over time and space.

Possible uses for this collection are limitless. Whether they be employed to teach a course in medical humanities, a translation project for students of Russian or French, or a project for a group of graphic design students, the posters have made their way into the University of Rochester curriculum. As curator of record for this collection, I have the opportunity to engage with classes, students, members of the press, and scholars. With each and every interaction I gain additional insights into how the messages and images can be grouped and arranged.

While we honored Dr. Atwater's request not to name the collection after him, we will always think of it as "his" collection. Though it continues to grow after losing him, the expansion of the collection is still very much tied to his vision and passion for collecting, and for documenting the social history of the ongoing AIDS crisis. Confident of the collection's continuing significance as a tool to understand the HIV/AIDS crisis from infinite perspectives, we know it will only become more important as we move through the twenty-first century and beyond. The kindness, generosity, and vision of Dr. Edward Atwater are at the heart of this collection. It is a deep privilege to build upon it and to share it with the world.

1   Dr. Edward C. Atwater, quoted by Hans Villarica, "30 Years of AIDS: 6,200 Iconic Posters, 100 Countries, 1 Collector," *The Atlantic*, Nov. 30, 2011, https://www.theatlantic.com/health/archive/2011/11/30-years-of-aids-6-200-iconic-posters-100-countries-1-collector/248737/ (accessed March 20, 2020).

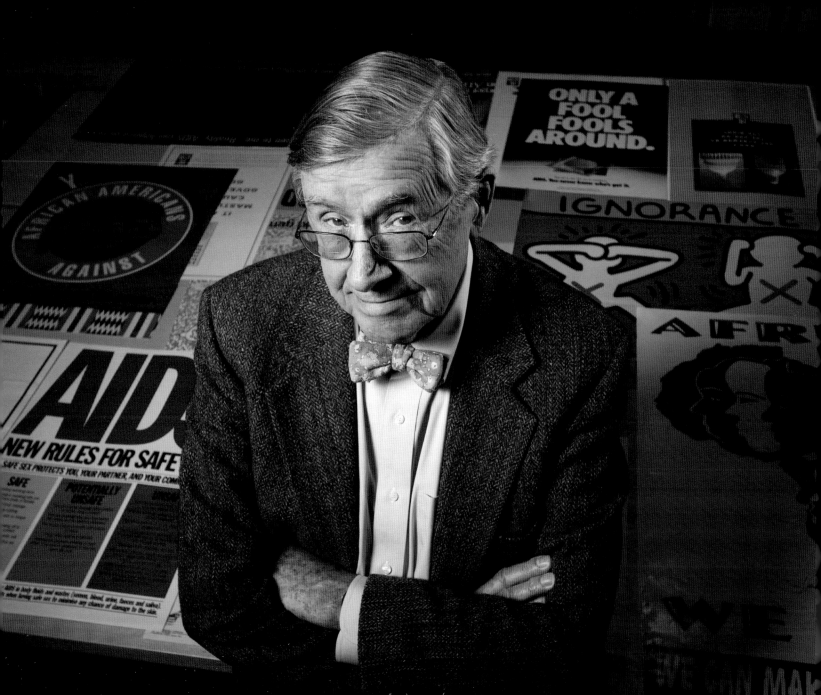

Afterword
Ending AIDS:
Or How to Manage an Epidemic

William M. Valenti, M.D.

Dr. Edward C. Atwater was no stranger to medical history, archiving, and documentation. As I have looked at parts of his collection over the years, sometimes at Ed's side, I see my patients—past and present. I have no doubt that the messages represented in the collection helped save many people's lives. I've learned something from each of these posters—about science, behavior, relationships, and the human condition, to name a few. More recently, though, I see the collection in a different way, as though I am seeing though a fresh pair of eyes. I see Ed Atwater's world view and a global chronology of the epidemic, which are foundational to the work ahead.

Shooting in the Dark
In June 1981, the first cases of what we now know as AIDS were reported by the Centers for Disease Control. They were described by my former medical student Dr. Michael Gottlieb. With that report, Gottlieb helped set the stage for exploring and defining a new disease. We had to make quick decisions about problems and issues that were previously unknown to us. We didn't realize it at the time, but we were, in fact, managing the epidemic. The "war zone" mentality of the era was overwhelming and traumatic, and it created a lasting impression. Nearly forty years later, one of our early nurses recalled, "There was death everywhere. We didn't even have time to mourn. We needed to get back to work."

Medical providers, health department staff, community organizations, advocates, educators, and artists partnered in response to this health crisis—an intersection of heavy doses of education and advocacy combined with the limited science of the time. The themes of the AIDS Education Posters collection follow the science and our understanding of AIDS from its emergence. Those themes loosely represent education, awareness, warnings, caution, contagion, behavior change, and safe(r) sex. The collection also chronicles the global response to the epidemic. At its core, it is the best representation anywhere of the early era of AIDS and its history.

Take, for example, Keith Haring's iconic "Ignorance = Fear. Silence = Death." This 1989 poster remains a call to action and continues to inspire me after all these years. Haring was an American artist who died of AIDS in 1990. His message? If we don't communicate effectively, we make no progress. Worse yet, if we fail to speak out, we have neglected our duty, as if we had done nothing at all.

In the 1980s and '90s, Haring's widely recognized graffiti-inspired figures championed AIDS education and compassion for the movement. The three figures with hands over their eyes, ears, and mouth represent the proverbial "See No Evil, Hear No Evil, Speak No Evil." This poster includes ACT UP's signature inverted pink triangle, a re-appropriation of the symbol that was used to identify gay people in Nazi concentration camps during World War II. ACT UP, the AIDS Coalition to Unleash Power, was founded in 1987 as a "diverse, non-partisan group of individuals united in anger and committed to direct action to end the AIDS crisis."[1] ACT UP's early acts of civil disobedience focused on increased federal funding for AIDS research, easing regulations to make HIV drugs available prior to final approval, and expanding funding for treatment and services for people living with HIV/AIDS.

The poster of a banana wearing a condom from the series *Banana Boys* (1983) (pages 154–155) was created by AIDS Rochester, the U.S. community service organization and a Trillium Health legacy organization. Like many organizations of the day, AIDS Rochester mobilized and made live presentations to health professionals, schools, community groups, and businesses. The poster represents a pivotal point in the movement. Condom discussions became *de rigueur,* and these educational sessions often included a health educator demonstrating how to put on a condom, the only prevention science we had at the time. We learned early that a banana worked best for visual effect and accuracy, even if it conflicted with some community standards. Otherwise the message would have been "Silence = Death." It also helped us stay on message that HIV is a sexually transmitted infection. One can't catch HIV from toilet seats, kissing, or casual contact.

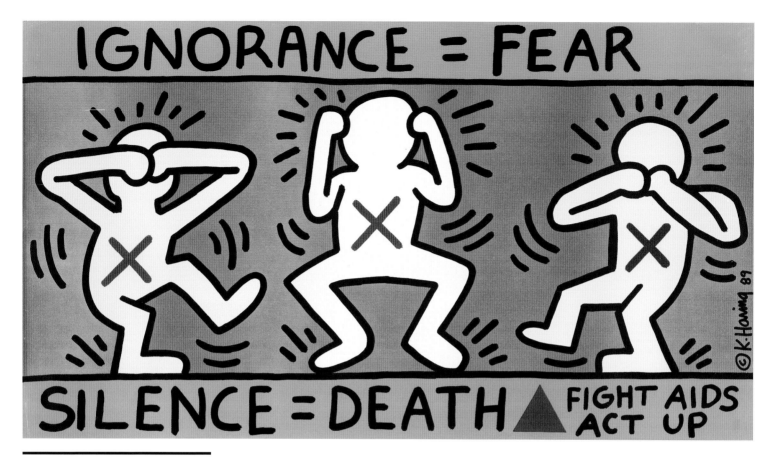

"Ignorance = Fear. Silence = Death," 1989
New York, New York, U.S.A.
Designer: Keith Haring
61 x 109 cm
AP6911

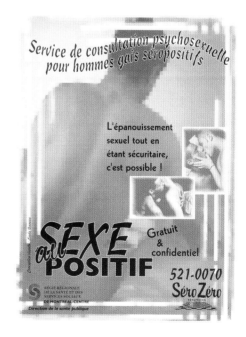

"Positive Sex," (translated from French),
1997
Montreal, Québec, Canada
Creator: Séro Zéro
Designer: Linda Daneau
62 x 45 cm
AP2485

"U = U," 2018
Atlanta, Georgia, U.S.A.
Creator: Centers for Disease Control
and Prevention/Division of HIV/AIDS
Prevention

"#PrEP4Sex," 2019
Rochester, New York, U.S.A.
Creator: Trillium Health Innovation Institute

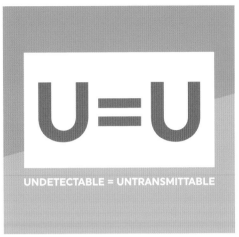

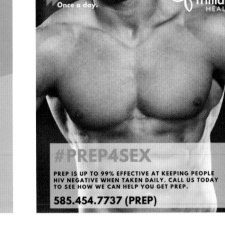

The name of that long-ago artist is lost. However, those of us who launched this campaign recall its inspiration as being Andy Warhol's album cover for the record *The Velvet Underground & Nico* (1967). A key historical document in the history of the AIDS epidemic, the banana image has flourished for years over print and digital media.

The 1997 poster "Sexe au positif" ("Positive Sex") was groundbreaking, in retrospect, and remains relevant all these years later. The poster, in French, from Québec Province's Ministry of Health and Social Services, offers counseling services for HIV-positive gay men. It speaks to sexual fulfillment while being safe. "It's Possible!" the poster states. This poster is an early Sex Positive effort—the social movement that takes a more accepting, enlightened view of sex, which diffuses stigma around sexual behavior.

Finishing the Job

The End the HIV Epidemic initiatives are built on the sacrifices of millions of people, their families, and communities whose lives were interrupted—a lost generation. If the past is prologue, the foundation laid by these sacrifices starting in 1981 has helped bring us to this point. AIDS was always a matter of urgency, and it is no different today. The End the HIV Epidemic movements taking place in New York and other states, the United States overall, and globally are equally urgent and compelling. All of these initiatives are designed to do one thing: stop the spread of HIV.

Today, the field of HIV Prevention Science builds on decades of accumulated evidence for both HIV treatment and prevention. The modern era Status Neutral approach can make ending the HIV epidemic a reality by interrupting HIV transmission.[2] Status Neutral programming is designed to stop HIV transmission, regardless of HIV status.

Those who are HIV positive are treated with antiretroviral drugs to achieve very low virus levels in their blood—a so-called "undetectable viral load"—so they do not spread the virus to others sexually. The Undetectable = Untransmittable (U =U) movement, promulgated by the poster above left, is now global and has been translated into hundreds of languages.

For HIV-negative people who are at risk, a new treatment is available called PrEP (HIV Pre-Exposure Prophylaxis). One pill a day is up to ninety-nine percent effective at preventing HIV infection. In the absence of a vaccine, biomedical HIV prevention will be taking center stage as injectable drugs, patches, and implants are in development and approved for use.

You Can't Send an Emoji or a Selfie on a Landline

Today people communicate, make friends, and arrange sexual encounters using mobile devices. How, then, do we translate the modern era's life-saving science into an understandable message? The people we need to reach are two or more generations away from the darkest days of AIDS and have no experience with the epidemic as it once was. The terms explosive, overwhelming, war zone, death sentence, fear of contagion, and the like are mere anecdotes to today's at-risk generation. The fear message doesn't work today, if it ever did.

As Avram Finkelstein states in the preface of this book, "the poster… will never become obsolete." In the early era of AIDS, the development of digital printing and composition changed the process of how posters were created. Now, the modern digital era presents another set of opportunities and challenges.

Today's messaging requires that we translate the subtle points of prevention science that can be viewed and understood on the screen of a smart phone, tablet, or even a smart wristwatch. A Trillium poster for PrEP (#PREP4SEX; above right) says it all. The image is sex positive, sells the product, and states the science succinctly. The image has appeared on posters and social media and can be read easily on a mobile device.

The emoji has also emerged as an educational and promotional tool geared to modern era communication (page 212). Trillium Health's PrEP emoji messaging can be viewed and understood on social media, smart phones, and other devices.

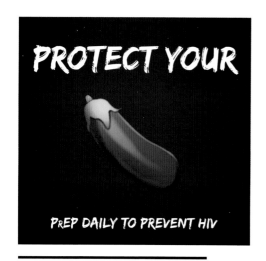

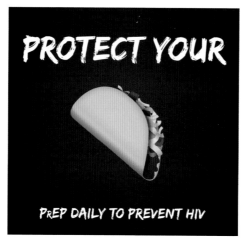

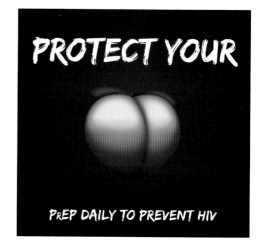

"Protect Your [Eggplant]," 2018
"Protect Your [Taco]," 2018
"Protect Your [Peach]," 2018
Rochester, New York, U.S.A.
Creator: Trillium Health Innovation
Institute Emoji Campaign

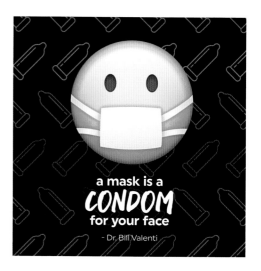

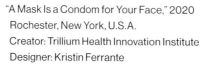

"A Mask Is a Condom for Your Face," 2020
Rochester, New York, U.S.A.
Creator: Trillium Health Innovation Institute
Designer: Kristin Ferrante

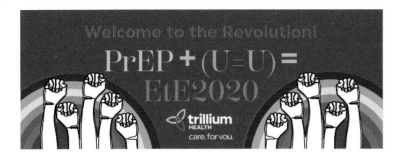

"Welcome to the Revolution!," 2018
Rochester, New York, U.S.A.
Creator: Trillium Health Innovation Institute
Designer: Joshua Elsenhemier

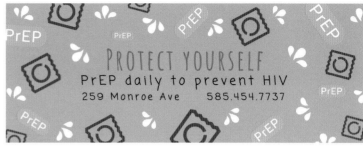

"Protect Yourself," 2018
Rochester, New York, U.S.A.
Creator: Trillium Health Innovation Institute

COVID-19: The Past is Prologue

The emergence of the COVID-19 pandemic adds additional strain on the End the HIV Epidemic initiatives. Trying to end one epidemic such as HIV during a global pandemic (COVID-19) is a major challenge.

The disruption of COVID-19 is reminiscent of the early "shooting in the dark" days of HIV; only more so. If the past is the prologue, critical decisions need to be made as the science of emerging infectious diseases evolves in spite of the unpredictable times.

Managing the HIV epidemic provides a blueprint for dealing with COVID-19, beginning with leadership at all levels of government, public health, and health care. Today, as in the past, posters and graphics continue to provide understandable information to vulnerable populations. COVID's themes are similar to those of HIV: the nuances of contagion, illness, economics, testing, legal matters, quarantine and isolation, and death. Like HIV, COVID-19 reminds us that people of color and marginalized populations remain vulnerable to infection.

Providing information on infection prevention is not a new concept. The difference is that the face mask and social distancing have replaced the condom as major prevention strategies.

In other words, the face mask is the COVID-19 pandemic's condom (page 212, bottom right)..

A World Without AIDS

We need to highlight End the HIV Epidemic initiatives in order to normalize HIV testing and the linkage to care, and to help stop the spread of HIV. Equally challenging is ensuring that these messages that connect with people on the screen of a smart phone also lend themselves to banners, rack cards, stickers, buttons, and pins.

The poster (above left) is an example of how to unify the modern era End the HIV Epidemic initiatives with the Status Neutral drivers of PrEP and U = U. In keeping with the past informing the future, note the homage to the earlier advocacy movement "Welcome to the Revolution!" The challenge is how to deliver the modern era message that speaks to HIV being "untransmittable" in patients taking HIV medications as described.

Another poster titled "Protect Yourself" (above right) shows it simply. The bold graphic engages the viewer. The text explains the science in two sentences. If repetition is the mother of learning, then PrEP and U = U will become universally acknowledged parts of the epidemic's management and its ultimate end.

Prevention Science redefines the condom in the contemporary era of End the HIV Epidemic, and the condom message is still relevant. In other words, Pre-Exposure Prophylaxis is more than taking one pill a day to prevent HIV. Using a sexual health framework, PrEP includes prevention, vaccinations, and screening and treatment

of sexually transmitted infections. Finally, the interactive nature of the digital format allows for "PrEP on demand" through online appointment scheduling and face-to-face medical appointments on a mobile device.

To end the HIV epidemic, our messaging must be grounded in contemporary HIV treatment and prevention science, be sex positive, and resonate with the reader. The message must also be versatile enough to be viewable and interactive either on a mobile device or when posted "Up Against the Wall."

Finally, now I can see a world without AIDS.

Notes

1. ACT UP's mission statement, https://actupny.com/contact/ (accessed March 25, 2020).
2. Camille Arkell, "An HIV Status Neutral Paradigm Shift," CatieBlog (November 4, 2019), "A status-neutral approach to HIV care means that all people, regardless of HIV status, are treated in the same way. It all starts with an HIV test. Any result, positive or negative, kicks off further engagement with the healthcare system, leading to a common final goal, where HIV is neither acquired nor passed," http://blog.catie.ca/2019/11/04/an-hiv-status-neutral-paradigm-shift/ (accessed March 25, 2020).

Contributors

Donald Albrecht is an independent curator and author based in New York City.

Jordan Arseneault is an artist, translator, and co-founder of the activist collective SéroSyndicat in Montréal.

Jonathan P. Binstock, Ph.D., is Mary W. and Donald R. Clark Director, Memorial Art Gallery, University of Rochester.

Ian Bradley-Perrin is a Ph.D. candidate in Sociomedical Sciences at Columbia University Mailman School of Public Health in New York City.

Jennifer Brier, Ph.D., is associate professor of gender, women's studies, and history at the University of Illinois at Chicago, where she also directs the program in gender and women's studies.

Tamar W. Carroll, Ph.D., is associate professor and chair, Department of History, Rochester Institute of Technology.

Mats Christiansen is a lecturer in nursing at Uppsala University, Sweden, and a Ph.D. candidate at Åbo Akademi University, Finland.

Siân Cook is a graphic designer and senior lecturer at London College of Communication.

Kyle Croft is programs manager at Visual AIDS in New York City.

Dr. Stephen Dewhurst is an HIV/AIDS researcher and the vice dean of research at the School of Medicine and Dentistry, University of Rochester.

Dr. Anthony S. Fauci is an immunologist and director of the National Institute of Allergy and Infectious Diseases.

Avram Finkelstein is a founding member of the Silence = Death and Gran Fury collectives.

Karen Herland is an activist, organizer, and educator currently teaching at Concordia University's Interdisciplinary Major in Sexuality Studies in Montréal.

Theodore (Ted) Kerr is a New York-based writer and a founding member of the collective What Would an HIV Doula Do?

Jessica Lacher-Feldman is exhibits and special projects manager and curator of the AIDS Education Posters collection at the University of Rochester, Department of Rare Books, Special Collections, and Preservation.

Dr. Joseph N. Lambert is an ophthalmologist in Irvine, California.

Mary Ann Mavrinac, Ed.D., is vice provost and Andrew H. and Janet Dayton Neilly Dean of the University of Rochester Libraries.

Alexander McClelland, Ph.D., who is living with HIV, is a Banting Postdoctoral Fellow, Department of Criminology at the University of Ottawa.

Esther McGowan is executive director of the nonprofit arts organization Visual AIDS.

Ken Monteith is executive director of COCQ-SIDA, the Québec coalition of AIDS organizations, based in Montréal.

Johnny Forever Nawracaj is a non-binary, Polish-born multidisciplinary artist who holds an MFA from Roski School of Art and Design at the University of Southern California in Los Angeles as well as an MA in art history from Concordia University in Montréal.

Joshua Valentine Pavan is co-founder of the Prisoner Correspondence Project, a solidarity project for queer prisoners in Canada and the United States, and outreach coordinator for the Support Staff Union at McGill University in Montréal.

MC Roodt is arts projects leader at the William Humphreys Art Gallery, an agency of the Department of Arts and Culture, South Africa, and chair for arts and health at the Public Health Association of South Africa.

Sur Rodney (Sur) is an independent archivist, curator, and writer in New York City and Montréal.

Dr. William M. Valenti is an infectious diseases specialist in Rochester, NY, and the co-founder of Community Health Network, now Trillium Health.

Matthew Wizinsky is a designer who runs the practice Studio Junglecat and is assistant professor at the University of Cincinnati's College of Design, Architecture, Art, and Planning.

Advisory Board

Acknowledgments

This book project relies heavily upon the people who have worked over the years to organize, digitize, and describe the collection of HIV/AIDS Education Posters. Among them are, of course, the donor and his spouse, Dr. Edward Atwater and Ruth Atwater, as well as their children, Ned Atwater and Rebecca Briccetti and their families.

Members of the River Campus Libraries team, including Clara AuClair, Lev Earle, Autumn Haag, Melissa Mead, Miranda Mims, Andrea Reithmayr, Marcy Strong, Jeff Suszczynski, Kristen Totleben, Melinda Wallington, and Lisa Wright, as well as former staff members including Lori Birrell and Jim Kuhn have worked on maintaining the physical and digital collection in the Department of Rare Books, Special Collections, and Preservation, River Campus Libraries, and have co-taught with the collection. Thanks to the work of Julia Maddox and Zoe Wisbey of the iZone in facilitating ideas around the title for the exhibition and book. We also acknowledge the numerous University of Rochester faculty and students who have used these posters in their own teaching and research, and to students who have worked with the posters, assisting in processing, access, and scholarship, including most recently, Katelyn Gibson, Miles Perry, and Jinxi Yu.

The project team working on every aspect of this major collaborative exhibition project includes Siri Baker, Stephanie Barrett, Sheri Burgstrom, Alyssa Bileschi, Jonathan Binstock, Nile Blunt, Rachael Brown, Joe Carney, Susie Daiss, Chris Garland, Jessica Gasbarre, Patti Giordano, Meredith Gozo, Pam Jackson, Travis Johansen, Mary Ann Mavrinac, Margot Muto, Eboni Jones Stewart, and Maurini Strub. Special thanks to the advisory board members, who have provided insights, ideas, and inspiration beyond measure.

Thank you to all of the chapter and section authors for sharing their knowledge and expertise. We acknowledge the efforts of Ian Bradley-Perrin. We are also deeply grateful to the team at RIT Press, to Ann Stevens, copyeditor, Dorie Jennings, proofreader, and to Rick Crummins at the University of Rochester for helping make the book a reality.

We are especially indebted to Dr. William Valenti, medical and consulting editor for this book, whose generosity, expertise, and compassion helped to bring this project to fruition.

Donald Albrecht acknowledges the efforts of Mark Resnick and especially Natalie Shivers in writing this book's introduction. Jessica Lacher-Feldman wishes to thank especially Dr. Edward Atwater and his family for the time, patience, and passion spent building this collection, and for the time spent together discussing the collection and more.

And finally, to the artists, designers, organizations, groups, and individuals who have expressed their words and images by creating these posters, and all of the posters in this collection, who have made their voices heard around the world. We thank you for your passion and compassion in fighting the global pandemic of HIV/AIDS.

Published and distributed by:
RIT Press
90 Lomb Memorial Drive
Rochester, NY 14623-5604
http://ritpress.rit.edu
Printed in the U.S.A.

Book and cover design: Marnie Soom
Typeface: Neue Haas Grotesk
Paper: Endurance Silk
Printing and binding: Shapco, Minneapolis, MN

ISBN 978-1-939125-78-1 (print)
ISBN 978-1-939125-79-8 (e-book)

Library of Congress Cataloging-in-Publication Data

Names: Albrecht, Donald, editor. | Lacher-Feldman, Jessica editor. |
    Valenti, William M., editor. | University of Rochester. Memorial Art
    Gallery, organizer, host institution.
Title: Up against the wall : art, activism, and the AIDS poster / edited by
    Donald Albrecht and Jessica Lacher-Feldman ; medical and consulting
    editor, William M. Valenti, M.D..
Other titles: Up against the wall (RIT Press)
Description: Rochester, NY : RIT Press, [2021] | Includes bibliographical
    references and index.
Identifiers: LCCN 2020045712 (print) | LCCN 2020045713 (ebook) | ISBN
    9781939125781 (hardcover) | ISBN 9781939125798 (ebook)
Subjects: LCSH: Public health posters—Exhibitions. | AIDS
    (Disease)—Posters—Exhibitions. | Atwater, Edward C.—Poster
    collections—Exhibitions. | Posters—New York
    (State)—Rochester—Exhibitions. | University of Rochester. River Campus
    Libraries—Poster collections—Exhibitions.
Classification: LCC NC1849.P78 U6 2021 (print) | LCC NC1849.P78 (ebook) |
    DDC 741.6/7409747—dc23
LC record available at https://lccn.loc.gov/2020045712
LC ebook record available at https://lccn.loc.gov/2020045713

Sponsored by Vicki and Richard Schwartz, the Rochester Area
Community Foundation's Lloyd E. Klos Fund, Friends of the University
of Rochester Libraries, DKT International, and the Gleason Family
Foundation. Additional support has been provided by the Family of Dr.
Edward C. Atwater, Helen H. Berkeley, Canandaigua National Bank and
Trust, the Gallery Council of the Memorial Art Gallery, the Anthony J.
Mascioli Trust, Suzanne M. Spencer, and an anonymous donor.

Funding is also provided by the Thomas and Marion Hawks Memorial
Fund, the Robert L. and Mary L. Sproull Fund, and the Nancy R. Turner
Fund for Special Exhibitions.

The exhibition is supported in part by awards from the National
Endowment for the Arts and the Institute of Museum and Library
Services MA-245369-OMS-20. The views, findings, conclusions
or recommendations expressed in this exhibition do not necessarily
represent those of the Institute of Museum and Library Services.

The book that complements the exhibition is made possible by
William M. Valenti, M.D., who served as medical and consulting editor
for the book project.

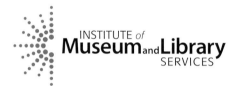

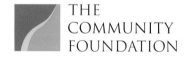

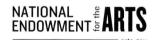

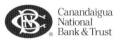